CENTRAL AUDITORY PROCESSING DISORDERS

Mostly Management

M. Gay Masters

State University of New York at Buffalo

Nancy A. Stecker

State University of New York at Buffalo

Jack Katz

State University of New York at Buffalo

D0082000

Allyn and Bacon

Boston • London • Toronto • Sydney • Tokyo • Singapore

Executive editor: Stephen D. Dragin
Series editorial assistant: Elizabeth McGuire
Manufacturing buyer: David Suspanic

Library of Congress Cataloging-in-Publication Data

Masters, M. Gay.
    Central auditory processing disorders: mostly management / M. Gay
Masters, Nancy A. Stecker, Jack Katz.
       p.   cm.
    Includes bibliographical references and index.
    ISBN 0-205-27361-0
    1. Word deafness--Treatment.   I. Stecker, Nancy Austin.
II. Katz, Jack. III. Title.
RC394.W63M37 1998
617.8--DC21   98-11753
                                    CIP
                                     Rev.

Printed in the United States of America
10 9 8 7 6 5 4 3 2 1   02 01 00 99 98

CONTENTS

PART II   *Management Approaches*

PART III   *Specific Methods and Populations*

LIST OF CONTRIBUTORS

Jane A. Baran, Ph.D.
Professor
Department of Communication Disorders
University of Massachusetts at Amherst
Amherst, Massachusetts

Brenda E. Berge, Au.D.
Private Practice
Washington, D.C.

Gail D. Chermak, Ph.D.
Professor and Chair
Department of Speech and Hearing Sciences
Washington State University
Pullman, Washington

Theresa M. Cinotti, M.A.
Assistant Clinical Professor
State University of New York at Buffalo
Speech-Language Pathologist
Buffalo Hearing and Speech Center
Buffalo, New York

Jeanane M. Ferre, Ph.D.
Audiologist, Private Practice
Oak Park, Illinois

Jack Katz, Ph.D.
Professor
Communicative Disorders and Sciences
State University of New York at Buffalo
Buffalo, New York

Warren D. Keller, Ph.D.
Psychologist, Private Practice
East Amherst Psychology Group
East Amherst, New York

M. Gay Masters, Ph.D.
Clinical Assistant Professor
Communicative Disorders and Sciences
State University of New York at Buffalo
Buffalo, New York

Larry Medwetsky, Ph.D.
Director of Audiology
Rochester Hearing and Speech Center
Rochester, New York

Frank E. Musiek, Ph.D.
Professor of Otolaryngology and Neurology
Director of Audiology
Dartmouth-Hitchcock Medical Center
Hanover, New Hampshire

Nancy A. Stecker, Ph.D.
Clinical Assistant Professor
Communicative Disorders and Sciences
State University of New York at Buffalo
Buffalo, New York

Ramona L. Stein, Ph.D.
Nu-Ear Hearing Aid Center, Inc.
Youngstown, Ohio

Kim L. Tillery, Ph.D.
Assistant Professor
State University of New York College at Fredonia
Fredonia, New York

Karen A. Yencer, Ph.D.
Audiologist, Private Practice
Amherst, New York

PREFACE

Numerous advances have been made in the area of assessment and management of central auditory processing disorders (CAPDs) over the past 10 years. In 1991, the Department of Communicative Disorders and Sciences at the State University of New York at Buffalo hosted a conference titled Central Auditory Processing: A Transdisciplinary View and published a book from the conference in 1992 by the same name. The purpose of the conference and book was to gather experts in the area of central auditory processing to discuss the anatomical and physiologic aspects, basic auditory processing considerations, and audiologic and speech-language approaches. Many requests were made for a follow-up conference with an emphasis on management. As a result, in September 1996, the State University of New York at Buffalo served as host for a conference titled Central Auditory Processing Disorders: Mostly Management. Again, experts from several professions were gathered to discuss issues regarding management of individuals with CAPDs. This book will provide the reader with updated information concerning CAPDs, as well as innovative management strategies.

This book is divided into three parts: Introduction (Chapters 1 through 3), Management Approaches (Chapters 4 through 8), and Specific Methods and Populations (Chapters 9 through 13). In Chapter 1, Stecker defines central auditory processing and describes the Buffalo Model of Central Auditory Processing Disorders. Musiek and Berge discuss the neurological underpinnings of auditory training and the role of plasticity in Chapter 2. They provide a neurologic justification for auditory therapy. In Chapter 3, Keller describes the relationship between attention deficit hyperactivity disorder (ADHD), central auditory processing disorders (CAPDs), and specific learning disorders. He also discusses the relationship between nonverbal learning disorders and other learning problems.

Part II emphasizes specific management approaches for CAPDs. In Chapter 4, Chermak describes metacognitive and metalinguistic approaches to managing CAPDs. Next, Medwetsky provides a basis for understanding memory and attention processing and associated management strategies in Chapter 5. Stein gives a detailed description in Chapter 6 of the use of FM technology in the classroom to aid those with CAPD. In Chapter 7, Ferre discusses an eclectic management approach to CAPD from the perspective of a private practice audiologist. She calls her management model M^3 and describes it in very practical terms. Masters concludes Part II by describing in Chapter 8 a speech-language approach to CAPD management. She gives a detailed explanation of the management strategies suggested in the Buffalo Model.

Innovative approaches and management techniques for special populations are described in Part III. In Chapter 9, Cinotti describes the new and innovative Fast ForWord program that strengthens temporal processing skills through the use of interactive software. Yencer discusses in Chapter 10 her results of a comprehensive investigation of the use of auditory integration therapy with children having CAPDs. Next, in Chapter 11, Tillery reports on management strategies and assessment approaches for those with CAPDs and ADHD. Baran describes management approaches for adolescents and adults with CAPDs in Chapter 12. She gives details of her program with college-age students with CAPDs. Finally, in Chapter 13, Katz describes the use of central auditory processing management strategies with cochlear implant users. He gives details of a specific phonemic approach that also could be beneficial to other groups with CAPDs.

ACKNOWLEDGMENTS

The authors would like to take this opportunity to thank many people for their support, understanding, and expertise throughout this process, from conference to book. We recognize the patience and love of our families: Irma Katz; Paul, Rachel, Emily, Andrew, and Jonathan Stecker; and Oksana Masters. Sandy Mundier is heartily thanked for her expertise in so many areas of our professional lives. Don Henderson originated the conference series in the Department of Communicative Disorders and Sciences, with the 1991 conference on central auditory processing disorders being the first of many successful conferences. Nancy Stecker, Jack

Katz, and Don Henderson contributed money from the 1991 conference to seed the 1996 conference on management of central auditory processing disorders. Start-up money for the 1996 conference was also provided by grants from Conferences in the Disciplines of the School of Social Sciences, State University of New York at Buffalo, and Conversations in the Disciplines, State University of New York. Our gratitude is also extended to the reviewers of this text, Susan M. Brander (Kean College of New Jersey) and Stephen T. Guryan (University of South Carolina), for their helpful comments. We also thank Jennifer Mackie for her assistance with the indexing.

Each of the contributing authors in this book patiently and promptly responded to every request, from the conference through the generation of the text. The many professionals in the public schools and other speech, language, and hearing clinics in western New York have challenged us to be clear and progressive in our diagnosis and management of central auditory processing disorders. The students of the Communicative Disorders and Sciences Department of the State University of New York at Buffalo have also helped us to grow in this area. Finally, we wish to thank the hundreds of clients with central auditory processing disorders and their families of the State University of New York at Buffalo Speech, Language, and Hearing Clinic, without whom none of this would have been possible.

1

OVERVIEW AND UPDATE OF CENTRAL AUDITORY PROCESSING DISORDERS

NANCY A. STECKER
State University of New York at Buffalo

In the broadest terms, *central auditory processing (CAP)* can be defined as "what we do with what we hear" (Katz, 1992). This phrase has been especially useful when describing CAP to parents and children. In March 1993, the American Speech-Language-Hearing Association (ASHA) brought together many professionals with expertise in CAP to discuss and reach consensus on a definition of central auditory processing. Experts also attempted to answer questions regarding basic science, assessment, developmental, and acquired communication problems relating to CAP. The report of the Task Force on CAP Consensus Development was published by ASHA in July 1996.

According to the Task Force, the definition of *central auditory processing* is the auditory system mechanisms and processes responsible for the following behavioral phenomena:

- Sound localization and lateralization
- Auditory discrimination
- Auditory pattern recognition
- Temporal aspects of audition, including
    Temporal resolution
    Temporal masking

Temporal integration
Temporal ordering
• Auditory performance decrements with competing acoustic signals
• Auditory performance decrements with degraded acoustic signals

The Task Force stated that these processes refer to verbal and nonverbal auditory signals that have neurophysiologic and behavioral correlates. *Central auditory processing disorders (CAPDs)* are defined as deficiencies in any one or more of these behaviors.

A multidisciplinary approach to CAPDs is suggested. To understand the process, one must take into account the physical nature of the acoustic stimulus, the neural mechanism that encodes the stimulus, the perceptual dimensions that arise from encoding, interactions between the perceptual and higher-level resources, and the nature of the pathological process (ASHA, 1996). Therefore, a team approach to assessment is preferred so that auditory performance deficits can be defined both thoroughly and functionally.

CAPD ASSESSMENT

The purpose of assessment is to (1) determine if CAPDs are present, (2) describe its parameters, and (3) indicate the functional effect of the auditory deficits. The assessment should consider the neuromaturational status of the auditory nervous system and should provide information about both developmental and acquired disorders.

Assessment often includes (1) a thorough history, (2) nonstandardized measures such as questionnaires or checklists concerning auditory behaviors, (3) behavioral and electrophysiologic test procedures, and (4) speech-language measures. The assessment measures should (1) be chosen by considering the chief complaint, (2) measure different central processes, (3) include both nonverbal and verbal stimuli, (4) be age appropriate, and (5) be reasonable in length (ASHA, 1996).

Peripheral assessment is an essential part of the CAPD battery and often includes pure tone thresholds, speech recognition, acoustic immittance measures and otoacoustic emissions (if available). Peripheral assessment must be included in the test battery to rule out hearing sensitivity loss and middle ear pathology. A history of conductive hearing loss was reported for 80 percent of all individuals referred for CAPD evaluations at the University at Buffalo Speech and Hearing Clinic.

The *behavioral CAP battery* could include tests of temporal processing, low-redundancy monaural speech, localization and lateralization, dichotic stimuli, and tests of binaural interaction. A comprehensive assessment is essential in order to develop an appropriate management plan for each individual. *Electrophysiologic measures* that could be part of the test battery include auditory brain stem response, as well as middle-, late-, and event-related evoked potentials. Chapter 2 gives an in-depth discussion regarding the use of electrophysiological tests for CAPD assessment.

THE BUFFALO MODEL

In order to better define CAPDs, Katz, Smith, and Kurpita (1992) described four clusters of test results and behavioral characteristics of those evaluated for CAPD. The four categories are decoding, tolerance-fading memory, integration, and organization. Each of the four categories has been associated with a specific region of the central nervous system (Katz, 1992). The four-category system has been particularly useful in diagnosing CAPDs as well as recommending appropriate management strategies.

In 1993, Masters, Stecker, and Katz presented the Buffalo Model of CAPD assessment and management. The model integrates the CAPD four-category system with the audiologic and speech-language evaluation results in order to prescribe an individual, comprehensive management plan. The model was developed to minimize overuse of labels and redundant recommendations that result from separate evaluations of those with CAPDs. By integrating test results of evaluators who consult on test outcomes and recommendations, a more appropriate and comprehensive management plan can be written.

The Buffalo Model includes a comprehensive audiological and speech-language assessment, as well as a thorough case history, an educational questionnaire completed by the teacher, and the Children's Auditory Processing Performance Scale (CHAPPS) (Smoski et al., 1992) completed by both the parents and teacher. At times, classroom observation of the child is included. The audiological assessment of this model always includes a comprehensive peripheral evaluation and a battery of CAPD measures. Pure tone air and bone conduction tests, speech thresholds, recorded word discrimination scores, otoscopy, tympanograms, ipsilateral and contralateral acoustic reflexes, and otoacoustic emissions are included in the peripheral assessment.

The CAP battery always includes the Staggered Spondaic Word (SSW) Test (Katz, 1986), the Phonemic Synthesis (PS) Test (Katz, 1983), a speech-in-noise (SN) test (Stecker, 1992), and the masking level difference (MLD) test (Stecker, 1992) at 500 Hz. Other tests are added as needed, such as the Auditory Continuous Performance Test (Keith, 1994), the Frequency Pattern Test (Musiek, 1994), the Duration Pattern Test (Musiek, 1994), compressed speech (Wilson et al., 1994) tests, and the Dichotic Digits (Noffsinger et al., 1994) Test. All tests are administered and scored according to standard procedures. Since the test battery is lengthy, breaks are given as needed.

The speech-language evaluation includes a comprehensive assessment of skills using measures such as a language sample, a word-finding test, a comprehension test, phonologic analysis, and other tests, as needed. Chapter 8 describes the speech-language measures in greater detail.

When the assessments are completed and all history and surveys have been received and reviewed, a conference with the family is held. During the conference, test results are reported, clarification questions are answered by both family members and evaluators, and possible recommendations are discussed. The child is included in the discussion as much as possible so that he or she understands the results and recommendations being made. Literature and handouts are available for distribution to families and schools for further information. Educational personnel are encouraged to contact the evaluators for further information concerning each individual assessed if needed. The Buffalo Model has been quite successful in developing comprehensive, individual management plans as well as helping families and educational personnel to better understand CAPDs.

CAPD CATEGORIES

The Buffalo Model uses the CAPD categories described by Katz, Smith, and Kurpita (1992) and expands to include speech-language test results and academic characteristics. The model combines results from the audiologic, speech-language, and educational evaluations to provide a more comprehensive, transdisciplinary profile of how an individual processes auditory information. Katz's research was based on observable clusters of test results and symptoms that seem to fall into distinct groups. The CAPD profiles help clinicians and others to better understand and predict areas of weakness, as well as to plan a more appropriate comprehensive management plan.

Decoding (DEC)

Decoding refers to the testing of those individuals who have difficulty in accurately and quickly processing what they hear. Individuals with weakness in this category have difficulty keeping up with the flow of communication, have poor phonemic skills, are slow responders, often have articulation errors (especially with /r/ and /l/), have difficulty following directions, and have weak oral reading and spelling skills. Their audiologic test results show "posterior" weakness signs on the SSW Test. It is very important to make note of qualitative information in addition to the quantitative test results. *Qualitative information* refers to test behaviors such as quick or slow responses on the SSW Test and repeating back the individual sounds on the Phonemic Synthesis Test (nonfused responses). A summary of this profile can be found in Table 1.1.

Often, the most valuable information for the CAP evaluation comes from how the individual handles the various tests, not just the scores on the tests. On the SSW Test, for example, those with decoding weaknesses often display a peak in the right competing and/or left noncompeting conditions, have long response delays, make more errors on the items presented to the right ear first, and make more errors on the second spondee compared to the first spondee. On the Phonemic Synthesis Test, these individuals have scores outside normal limits for their grade level and have delayed and sometimes nonfused responses. A speech-in-noise deficit is sometimes present.

Speech-language test results for an individual with decoding difficulties often shows weak receptive language skills, articulation errors, word-finding problems, prosody errors, and problems with oral and written discourse (see Chapter 8).

TABLE 1.1   Decoding Profile

Audiological Findings	Speech-Language Findings	Academic Implications
History of conductive HL	Receptive language: morphology	Slow responder

SSW
  Right competing, left
    noncompeting peak
  Order effect L/H
  Ear effect H/L
	Word-finding errors
	
	Prosody errors
		Phonics problems:
		  Reading
		  Spelling

PS
  Nonfused delays
  < grade expectations
	Discourse: oral and
	  written
		Poor understanding of
		  directions
		Weak on written tests
		Minimal oral discussions

SN
  Mild to moderate
    difficulty (score in
    quiet minus score in
    noise)
	Articulation errors:
	  /r/ & /l/
		Difficulty with group
		  listening

Tolerance-Fading Memory (TFM)

Tolerance-fading memory is characterized by those people who have difficulty understanding speech under adverse conditions and who also display short-term memory weaknesses. Although some individuals will
show weakness in only one of these areas, it is most common for both
conditions to be present, especially in severe cases. Katz's (1992) research
shows that the anterior temporal region and frontal lobes are responsible
for these skills. Individuals experiencing TFM typically are impulsive
responders, are easily overstimulated, and may be hyperacusic. They
also typically have poor reading comprehension skills and handwriting
due to poor motor planning, have short attention spans, and are easily
distracted.

   Those displaying a TFM type of CAPD often exhibit similar characteristics to those with attention deficit disorder (ADD) and attention deficit hyperactivity disorder (ADHD). It is suggested that the Auditory
Continuous Performance Test (ACPT) be administered if ADD or ADHD
is suspected (Tillery, 1997). This test screens for attention disorders and
can be used as part of a CAPD test battery to aid in differential diagnosis
and lead to appropriate referral for further assessment by a neuropsychologist. For further discussion of ADHD, see Chapters 3 and 11.

   Audiologic test results that are typically displayed with individuals
who have a TFM type of CAPD include a peak in the left competing condition on the SSW Test. Qualitatively, they often are very impulsive
responders, which leads to more errors on the first spondee heard, and
also tend to err on items presented to the left ear first. These individuals
will often have difficulty on items that are referred to as tongue twisters
(i.e., they get tangled up in saying their responses). Two words may be
combined so that a new word that was not presented is in the response.
For example, on the item *bedspread-mushroom,* they might respond *bed
spushroom.* On the Phonemic Synthesis Test, there are usually qualitative
signs such as omitting initial sounds and quick, impulsive responses.
Speech-in-noise test results are usually significantly below expected levels. Often, these individuals display great anxiety during this procedure,
are quite fidgety, and show considerable struggle.

   Speech-language findings include expressive language problems
and sometimes cluttering. Articulation skills in isolated words are usually normal but in connected discourse are often inconsistent, with
coalescent- and metathesis-type errors. Receptive language skills are
weak when elaborated syntax is assessed. Individuals displaying TFM
often have a reduced ability to make inferences and show short-term
memory weaknesses. The TFM profile is summarized in Table 1.2.

TABLE 1.2   Tolerance-Fading Memory Profile

Audiological Findings	Speech-Language Findings	Academic Implications

SSW
  Left competing
      peak
  Order effect H/L
  Ear effect L/H
  Smushes, too
    quick, tongue
    twisters
 	
PS
  Omits first sounds
 	
S/N
  >40% discrepancy
    from quiet WDS
 	
Hyperacusis
	Expressive language
	  weakness: cluttering
	Inconsistent articulation:
	  Coalescence
	  Metathesis
	Receptive language
	  weakness:
	  elaborated syntax
	Discourse errors: oral and
	  written
		Poor attention span
		Distractible
		Reading weaknesses:
		  Comprehension
		  Inferences
		Weak short-term memory
		Following directions
		Poor handwriting
		Impulsive
		Poor motor planning

Integration (INT)

Integration refers to the characteristics seen in individuals who have difficulty integrating auditory information with other functions, such as visual or nonverbal aspects of speech. There are two subtypes in this category: INT Type 1, which is similar to the decoding profile, and INT Type 2, which is similar to the TFM profile. However, INT cases display more severe problems than the DEC and TFM profiles and have a specific test pattern. Katz (1992) states that the corpus collosum and the angular gyrus are associated to the weaknesses seen in the INT profile. Individuals displaying INT are usually learning disabled, very poor readers, and often labeled as dyslexic. The INT Type 1 profile also includes very poor spelling skills, poor sound-symbol relationships, excessively slow response rate, and very poor handwriting. These individuals also are often poor at multimodal tasks, including using appropriate affect with speech.

Audiologic test results of both Type 1 and 2 include a type A pattern on the SSW Test. This is a particular cluster of errors that has been associated with severe reading and spelling disorders (Katz & Ivey, 1993). Qualitatively, individuals experiencing this condition usually have extremely long delays in responding. On the Phonemic Synthesis Test, those with Type 1 signs score below expected grade level, display long delays and nonfused responses, and often quietly rehearse their answers before responding. Speech-in-noise test results are very poor in those with Type 2 INT and will sometimes show a large discrepancy between the two ear scores. It is advised to include a binaural presentation of this test as well as monaural presentations to assess the integration between the ears.

Speech-language test results show word-finding problems. Receptive language weaknesses noted in those with INT-type profiles include morphological and syntactical errors. Expressive language weaknesses are noted in both oral and written discourse. The INT profile is summarized in Table 1.3.

Organization (ORG)

Organization is characterized by reversals and sequencing errors. Individuals experiencing this condition are often quite disorganized at school and at home (Lucker, 1981). This profile usually is secondary to another CAPD category and is rarely evident in isolation of another CAPD profile. These individuals display reversals on audiologic and speech-language tests. Errors in listener perspective are sometimes evident in discourse. The ORG profile is summarized in Table 1.4.

Multiple Categories

Most individuals who are seen for CAP evaluations demonstrate weaknesses in more than one category. Usually, the categories displayed are

TABLE 1.3   Integration Profile

Audiological Findings	Speech-Language Findings	Academic Implications

SSW
   Type A
   Sharp left competing
      peak
   Extreme delays
PS
   < grade expectations
   Nonfused delays
   Quiet rehearsals
S/N
   Discrepancy between
      ears
	Word-finding problems
	Receptive language
	   errors:
	   Morphology
	   Syntax
	Expressive language
	   errors: oral and
	   written
		Extremely slow
		   responder
		Poor phonetic skills
		Poor sound-symbol
		   relationships
		Severe reading and
		   spelling problems
		Very poor handwriting
		Difficulty with multi-
		   modal tasks

TABLE 1.4   Organization Profile

Audiological Findings	Speech-Language Findings	Academic Implications
SSW	Discourse errors: oral and written	Sequencing errors
Reversals	Sequencing	Disorganized in work
PS	Listener perspective	
Reversals		

ranked by severity as primary, secondary, or tertiary. There is often agreement between speech-language and audiologic test results when assessing CAP abilities. Although there is often agreement in diagnosing CAPDs, there is considerable value in carrying out both evaluations when planning management strategies. The ASHA (1996) Consensus Task Force strongly recommended both audiologic and speech-language evaluations be carried out in making a CAPD diagnosis.

In 1993, Masters, Stecker, and Katz presented data on 25 children referred for CAPD evaluations. A comprehensive audiologic and speech-language evaluation was carried out on each child. Of the total, 1 child was found to be within normal limits on both audiologic and speech-language batteries; 23 children were diagnosed as having significant CAPD on both batteries. The speech-language pathologist reported decoding as the primary CAPD category for 18 children and tolerance-fading memory as primary for 5 children. The audiologist reported 15 children having decoding as the primary category and 8 with tolerance-fading memory as the primary category. Significant tolerance-fading memory difficulties on the audiologic tests were experienced by 1 other child but the speech-language tests were within normal limits. This is probably reflective of the different stimuli used and areas tested by the two professions administering the tests.

Similar data were collected from 1995 and 1996 at the Speech-Language and Hearing Clinic at the University at Buffalo. Over 300 subjects were assessed. Again, there was significant agreement between speech-language and audiologic test results; all cases were diagnosed as having CAPDs by both professions. Of the 300 children, 49 percent showed primary decoding profiles, 43 percent showed primary tolerance-fading memory profiles, and 8 percent showed primary integration profiles. Secondary and tertiary signs by percentage can be found in Table 1.5. These results were in close agreement with those of Katz (1992). It is also worth noting that 80 percent of the 300 children had a significant history of conductive hearing loss.

TABLE 1.5   CAPD Profile Data of 300 Children (in Percent)

Category	Primary	Secondary	Tertiary	Total
Decoding	49% (146)	16% (24)	4% (1)	69%
Tolerance-fading memory	43% (130)	23% (35)	9% (2)	73%
Integration	8% (24)	0	0	8%
Organization	0	14% (21)	4% (1)	18%
	100% (300)	53% (80)	17% (4)	

MANAGEMENT STRATEGIES BY CAPD PROFILE

The Buffalo Model not only divides CAPDs into four categories but it also recommends management strategies that are most appropriate for the four profiles. This is probably the greatest beneficial use of the category system in CAPD assessment. Table 1.6 summarizes intervention strategies for each category and are further described in other chapters in this book.

Decoding

The management strategies for *decoding* difficulties center on improvement of phonemic and metaphonolgical skills. A phonetic approach to reading instruction is advised. All auditory information and directions should be presented in a clear and concise manner. Rephrasing and restating oral directions is often necessary, as well as frequent repetition. Pretutoring of academic material is suggested for the classroom, and outlines of new topics and written instructions for those who can read are helpful. Chapter 7 describes specific phonemic tasks that have proved to be successful with those who fall into this decoding profile. Chapter 8 describes several useful strategies for improving auditory decoding skills. Bellis (1996) suggests that management strategies for those with decoding weaknesses are similar to those suggested for traditional aural rehabilitation.

Tolerance-Fading Memory

Tolerance-fading memory management strategies focus on improving the signal-to-noise ratio and strengthening short-term memory skills. Improving the signal-to-noise ratio can be accomplished by changing the acoustic environment of the classroom, seating the child close to the

TABLE 1.6 Intervention Strategies

Audiological/Speech Language	Academic
Decoding	
Improve phonemic and metaphonological skills: Phonemic Synthesis Program Auditory Discrimination in Depth Hooked on Phonics Rhyming, syllable, and phoneme segmentation	Reading: Phonetic approach Directions: Clear, concise, and repeated Testing modifications Outlines Rephrase and restate Pretutoring Written instructions
Tolerance-Fading Memory	
Improve the signal-to-noise ratio: Assistive listening device Alter classroom acoustics Noise desensitization practice Compensatory strategies for auditory memory: Identify classroom scripts Rehearsal strategies Imposing a delay Teach outlining and notetaking Mnemonics and chunking	Preferential seating Earplugs Obtain attention: Eye contact Call name Gentle touch Take notes and outline Tape record classes Quiet study areas
Integration	
Improve phonemic and metaphonological skills Improve signal-to-noise ratios	Note-takers Tape record classes Reader-writer for tests Texts on tape Word processor with audio spell-check
Organization	
Discourse therapy: sequence, information	Consistent routines Checklists, calendar

teacher, and using assistive listening devices. The use of FM auditory training devices in the classroom has been shown to provide significant benefit to some children. Chapter 6 discusses this approach in detail.

Noise desensitization training has also been shown to be beneficial. This approach involves exposing the individual to a noise while carrying out another task. The noise is gradually increased as the individual becomes more efficient at listening during the noise. The type of noise used can also be varied, from music to a single speaker in the background. The objective is to desensitize the individual to noise and to build a greater tolerance to noise. Other management strategies include use of earplugs and quiet study areas. Employing compensatory strategies for short-term memory, tape recording classes, and using a note-taker are often recommended. Chapter 5 describes a systematic approach for improving memory skills.

Integration

Integration management strategies focus on improving phonemic and metaphonologic skills. A very structured, phonetic approach to reading instruction is suggested, such as the Orton-Gillingham method. Compensatory strategies include using note-takers, reader/writer for tests, and books on tape, and tape recording lectures. A word processor with an audio spell-check can also be useful. Improving the signal-to-noise ratio is often necessary. Bellis (1996) suggests activities that improve interhemispheric transfer of information for individuals with this profile. These include use of visual, tactile, and somatasensory aids along with auditory tasks. Music training, dancing, and singing have been suggested as good interhemispheric tasks.

Organization

Management strategies to improve *organization* skills usually focus on improving sequencing skills and organizational habits. Discourse therapy for sequencing of information is described in Chapter 8. Following consistent routines at school and home are essential. Use of checklists, appointment books, and calendars is also suggested. Chapter 4 describes metacognitive tasks that could be beneficial for those with organizational weaknesses.

SUMMARY

This chapter has provided the reader with a background of some basic principles of CAP and CAPDs. Two definitions of CAPDs were given. One is simply "what we do with what we hear" (Katz, 1992) and the other is the ASHA Task Force on CAP definition. The later definition gives the clinician a comprehensive, detailed model of CAP, whereas the first provides an easy, practical explanation for those not familiar with CAP. The ASHA Task Force on CAP Consensus Development statement was summarized, including assessment and management suggestions. The four-category system to CAPD was described, as well as the Buffalo Model to CAPD assessment and management.

REFERENCES

American Speech-Language-Hearing Association. (1996, July). Central auditory processing: Current status of research and implications for clinical practice. *American Journal of Audiology, 5*, 2.

Bellis, T. J. (1996). *Assessment and management of central auditory processing disorders in the educational setting from science to practice.* San Diego: Singular Publishing Group.

Katz, J. (1983). Phonemic synthesis. In E. Lasky & J. Katz (Eds.), *Central auditory processing disorders: Problems of speech, language and learning* (pp. 540–563). Baltimore: University Park Press.

Katz, J. (1986). *The SSW manual* (3rd ed.). Vancouver, WA: Precision Acoustics.

Katz, J. (1992). Classification of auditory processing disorders. In J. Katz, N. Stecker, & D. Henderson (Eds.), *Central auditory processing: A transdisciplinary View.* St. Louis: Mosby.

Katz, J., & Ivey, R. (1993). Spondaic procedures in central testing. In *Handbook of clinical audiology.* Baltimore: Williams and Wilkins.

Katz, J., Smith, P., & Kurpita, B. (1992). Categorizing test findings in children referred for auditory processing defits. *SSW Reports, 14*, 1–6.

Keith, R. (1994). *Auditory Continuous Performance Test, examiner's manual.* San Antonio: Harcourt Brace.

Lucker, J. (1981). Interpreting SSW results of learning disabled children. *SSW News, 3*, 1–3.

Masters, M., Stecker, N., & Katz, J. (1993, November). *CAP disorders, language difficulty, and academic success: A team approach.* Presented at the American Speech-Language-Hearing Association Convention, Los Angeles.

Musiek, F. (1994). Frequency (pitch) and duration pattern tests. *Journal of the American Academy of Audiology, 54*, 265–268.

Noffsinger, D., Martinez, C., & Wilson, R. (1994). Dichotic listening to speech: Background and preliminary data for digits, sentences, and nonsense syllables. *Journal of the American Academy of Audiology, 5*, 248–254.

Smoski, W., Brunt, M., & Tannahill, J. (1992). Listening characteristics of children with central auditory processing disorders. *Language, Speech and Hearing Services in the Schools, 23*, 145–152.

Stecker, N. (1992). Audiologic considerations and approaches. In J. Katz, N. Stecker, & D. Henderson (Eds.), *Central auditory processing: A transdisciplinary view* (pp. 117–126). St. Louis: Mosby.

Tillery, K. (1997). *A double-blind study of the central auditory processing and auditory continuous performances of children with attention deficit hyperactivity disorder and central auditory processing disorder under ritalin and placebo conditions.* Unpublished doctoral dissertation, State University of New York at Buffalo.

Wilson, R., Preece, J., Salamon, D., Sperry, J., & Bornstein, S. (1994). Effects of time compression plus reverberation on the intelligibility of Northwestern University Auditory Test No. 6. *Journal of the American Academy of Audiology, 5*, 269–277.

2

A NEUROSCIENCE VIEW OF AUDITORY TRAINING/ STIMULATION AND CENTRAL AUDITORY PROCESSING DISORDERS

FRANK E. MUSIEK
Dartmouth-Hitchcock Medical Center

BRENDA E. BERGE
Private Practice

The concept of auditory training (AT) dates back to the sixth century. Initially, AT was used with individuals who had severe hearing loss, probably of peripheral origin. The logic behind early AT was that if one practiced listening to different sounds, overall hearing would improve. For many years, auditory training was implemented in schools for the deaf and in rehabilitation clinics. At one time (after World War II), it was relatively common to have most hearing-aid users undergo some type of AT. However, due to a lack of a good scientific base, lack of clinical efficacy, and general lack of interest in the professional community, AT became a seldom used therapeutic procedure in audiology.

Recently, AT has been revived, but not so much for use with peripheral hearing loss but rather for those with central auditory processing disorders (CAPD). Conversely to the early days of AT, there are currently strong neuroscience underpinnings that are the driving force behind AT, supporting its use with CAPD. Recent reports, which will be discussed later, have shown improvement in certain auditory tasks after acoustic stimulation and training. These improvements in performance certainly are not related to alteration of the auditory periphery but rather the central auditory nervous system (CANS).

The plasticity of the CANS is the key factor in the improvements shown through AT and auditory stimulation. It seems as though the amount of plasticity increases in caudal to rostral progression in the auditory system. This notion may also be related to the idea that improvement in auditory function is greater when the task measured is complex rather than simple. For example, it is well known that AT will not improve a simple task such as pure tone thresholds, yet more complex tasks such as pattern perception or speech tasks appear to improve with appropriate training (Gengel & Hirsh, 1970; Neisser & Hirst, 1974).

One of the best examples of improvement of auditory function with training comes from observations made on World War II Morse code operators. These individuals had to discriminate acoustic patterns that were often buried in noise. They were highly motivated people because a great deal hinged on whether they could understand the often garbled code. It was well known that experienced Morse code operators were able to decipher messages that untrained personnel could not begin to understand. However, with training, novel code interpreters became very adept at the task.

REVIEW OF AUDITORY TRAINING/STIMULATION

Wedenberg (1951) traced the early history of auditory training and found that in the sixth century, doctors used large bells in an attempt to stimulate hearing in the deaf. In the 1800s, Itard, at the Paris School for the Deaf, is credited with teaching auditory identification of vowels and consonants, as well as high- versus low-pitched sounds to his students (Hudgins, 1954). Itard reported subsequent improvements in communication of his students on this AT program (Hudgins, 1954). In England, Toynbee in the 1860s and Urbantschitch in the 1890s both embellished on Itard's AT approach and reported successes in many of their clients (Wedenberg, 1951). Max Goldstein, who founded the Central Institute for the Deaf, studied with Urbantschitch and brought many AT methods to the United States around 1930. According to Wedenberg, Forester in 1928 and Goldstein in 1936 performed similar studies that showed AT did not improve pure tone thresholds but did improve speech understanding.

A major contribution at the time was DiCarlo's (1948) book on AT, which emphasized discrimination of speech sounds. Later, efforts that focused AT on identification and discrimination of rhythmic patterns, melodies, isolated phonemes, letters, and digits, and minimally different words as well as frequency and intensity discrimination seemed to advance the field in a more sophisticated, scientific direction (DiCarlo, 1948; Huizing, 1952; Kelly, 1954; Carhart, 1960; Doehring & Ling, 1971). Sanders (1971) wrote about high and low redundancy AT—that is, training in ideal listening conditions versus training in challenging acoustical situations and on demanding tasks.

The more recent approaches to AT can be placed into several categories (Blamey & Alcantara, 1994). The *analytic* approach, similar to approaches mentioned earlier, attempts to break speech into components (e.g., phonemes) that serve as the basis for AT. The *synthetic* approach is therapy that uses clues from context and syntax to help derive meaning. The *pragmatic* approach has the listener control communication factors such as intensity, signal-to-noise ratio, and so on. The *eclectic* approach is defined by combining several of the AT procedures just mentioned.

One of the recent methods for AT with children has been described by Erber (1982). This method requires the use of the Glendonald Auditory Screening Procedure (GASP) assessment battery, which takes into account the complexity of the speech signal and the form of response from the listener. The Erber approach is highly adaptable to many levels of auditory abilities because stimulus-response can range from simple to complex (Schow & Nerbonne, 1996).

The DASL (Developmental Approach to Successful Listening) consists of a sequential, structured program that emphasizes a hierarchy of listening skills (Stout & Windle, 1992). A newer approach to consonant recognition training has been reported by Walden and colleagues (Walden et al., 1981). This approach was shown to improve consonant recognition and the perception of sentences in a combined auditory and visual therapy methodology.

The forementioned review of AT, though showcasing a variety of methods, did have one factor in common: The patients/clients had hearing loss (presumed peripheral hearing loss). In the 1970s and 1980s, AT expanded to include patients with cochlear implants and individuals with CAPD. The CAPD group often complained of difficulty hearing but demonstrated normal audiograms. It is this group that will be discussed in more detail in this chapter. With the patients with CAPD, the AT is directed more toward central mediated functions of hearing and language, although some of the same approaches mentioned earlier may also be worthwhile.

Phonemic synthesis, introduced in 1982, centered on blending sounds into words (Katz & Harmon, 1982). This technique reportedly improved phonemic synthesis ability and increased decoding skills on the Lindamood Auditory Conceptualization (LAC) test (Katz, 1983). Alexander and Frost (1982) reported on AT with decelerated speech that was time expanded 60–80 msec. for transitions. This technique showed improvement in discrimination for children with language delays. Tallal and associates (1996) used a similar AT paradigm as Alexander and Frost but the former used a 50 percent time expansion and enhanced the "fast" transitional elements by 20 dB. This approach also showed improvement in children with language learning impairments.

Sloan (1986) published a thorough, systematic approach to AT for CAPD that emphasized speech sound discriminations alone, in combinations, and in context. Chermak and Musiek (1992) and Musiek and Chermak (1995) outlined a variety of AT approaches to use with children with CAPD, including recommendations on prosodic and intonation features. Tallal and colleagues (1996) and Merzenich and colleagues (1996) showed improvement in the temporal ordering of acoustic elements (speech segments and complex tones) by adaptive training on temporal ordering tasks.

Auditory training/stimulation for CAPD has gained interest and respect recently, not only due to different techniques and approaches that are available but also because neuroscience has provided evidence that functional and microstructural changes in the brain evolve with appropriate training/stimulation. It also has become evident that without stimulation and training, the CANS maybe compromised. The next section of this chapter will focus on some of the critical advances in understanding both stimulation and deprivation of the CANS. These advances, linked to plasticity, provide direction and concepts key to auditory training for CAPD and related communicative problems.

KEY CNS FUNCTIONS AND AUDITORY TRAINING/STIMULATION

Plasticity

One key factor related to improvement from audio training is neural plasticity. Lund (1978) defines *neural plasticity* as "neural form and connections that take on a predictable pattern (probably genetically determined) often referred to as neural specificity; exceptions to this predictable pattern, in certain circumstances, represents neural plasticity" (p. 5). We propose another definition: The alteration of nerve cells to better conform to immediate environmental influences, with this alteration often associated with behavioral change. There are three general types of plasticity:

developmental, compensatory (after lesions or damage), and learning related (Scheich, 1991). Auditory enhancement through AT for CAPD could involve all three types of plasticity.

If neural plasticity is a change in nerve cells due to environmental influences, and if one can control and shape those influences in a desired manner, one might predict the behavior related to the plasticity. In a model, AT could be viewed as the environmental influence, and nerve cells in the CANS could represent the associated neural change. In neural plasticity, as the environment (acoustic stimuli) is altered, associated changes in the CANS nerve cells take place. Perhaps one of the best ways to further discuss neural plasticity, the CANS, and AT is to focus on relevant areas of plasticity for which there is considerable documentation. Three areas of plasticity for which there is fairly good documentation relevant to AT is long-term potentiation (LTP), auditory deprivation, and auditory stimulation.

Long-Term Potentiation

Long-term potentiation (LTP) has commonly been associated with the physiologic basis of learning and memory, but it may not be limited to these processes. Hebb (1949) suggested that the basic mechanisms of learning and memory were due to modifications of neural tissue from pre- and poststimulus activity of neurons. These modifications were thought to be related to growth of novel connections in the brain. Support for this idea came from demonstrations that showed functional changes that occurred in neurons were a direct result of their repetitive use. These changes are an increase in the strength of synaptic transmission. When the increased strength lasts for more than minutes, this form of plasticity is referred to as LTP (Greenough & Bailey, 1988).

Early theorists in neuroscience believed that plasticity could occur throughout the life span; early experimental results did not support this position, however. It was commonly thought that one could not bring about changes in the CNS with practice or stimulation. This notion carried over to many of the clinical disciplines, including audiology. It was this lack of scientific support that decreased interest in AT in the 1960s through 1990s. However, in 1964, Rosenzweig, Bennett and Krech demonstrated that rats reared in visually complex environments had a greater volume of occipital cortex than those reared in cages. The implication was that adult brains could be altered through stimulation enhancement. Though this study and the concepts associated with it came under much scrutiny and controversy, it spawned further scientific interest in LTP. From a number of these studies some important concepts of LTP were formed. Since this early research, it has been learned that

LTP occurs whether the repeated stimulus was sensory or electrical and that the LTP can last for long durations (i.e., weeks/months)—especially if the stimulus trains are of greater strength (Bliss & Lomo, 1973; Bliss & Gardner-Medwin, 1973; Bailey & Chen, 1988).

Relevant to the auditory system, Rogan and LeDoux (1995) applied electrical and then auditory stimulation to the medial geniculate body. They found that LTP occurred to the acoustic stimulus in a neural tract coursing from the medial geniculate body to the amygdala. This finding was important because it demonstrated that naturally occurring stimuli could result in LTP and that sensory (auditory) tissue can respond in this manner.

Clearly, the concept of repetition resulting in LTP has implications to all sensory and cognitive systems in terms of stimulation and training. Long-term potentiation appears to be a physiologic correlate to an apparent neural conditioning that many scientists believe is linked to memory or learning. It is interesting that the time course of LTP, as well as the way in which variations in the stimulus can change LTP duration, seem to be similar to memory findings (Lund, 1978). Also of special interest is that the LTP neurons (which are cortical or subcortical) are different from peripheral sensory neurons, which adapt with rapid stimulations instead of increasing their response strength.

In LTP, stimulation is the key factor related to plasticity. Without stimulation, whether it be natural or artificial, LTP cannot take place. When a system that is stimuli responsive does not receive stimulation, deprivation takes place. The effects of deprivation, specifically sensory deprivation, have not been well understood until recently. This area of study has also become a popular area of neuroscience.

Auditory Deprivation

Auditory deprivation can result in various forms of plasticity. When physiological systems that are designed to respond primarily to stimulation are not stimulated, the neural system changes. Many pioneers in the early use of AT realized that the auditory system was not stimulated sufficiently, hence they tried various ways to stimulate it. More recently, scientists have demonstrated what happens to the auditory system when it is deprived of sufficient sound stimulation.

There are a variety of ways in which deprivation has been achieved in animals, with the results being determined by anatomical, physiological, or behavioral measures. Interestingly, regardless of the manner of deprivation or the type of outcome measure, the results are similar.

Webster (1977; Webster & Webster, 1983) showed that auditory deprivation accomplished by sound isolation resulted in the reduction of cell volumes of auditory structures in the low brain stem. Experimentally induced conductive hearing losses in animals have also shown anatomic or physiologic effects on central auditory structures in the brain stem (Evans, Webster, & Cullen, 1983; Webster, 1983, 1988; Clopton & Silverman, 1978). Clearly, conductive losses early in life seem to delay appropriate maturation of brain stem auditory nuclei (Evans et al., 1983; Webster, 1983; Walger et al., 1993). Cochlear damage that results in hearing loss has also been linked to (transynaptic) degeneration of the auditory nuclei and associated fibers in the brain stem (Morest, 1983; Hall, 1976; Tucci et al., 1987). Early cochlear damage secondary to noise exposure has also been shown to manifest as poor tonotopic organization at the inferior colliculus (Pierson & Synder-Keller, 1994).

A different result from noise damage to the cochlea was reported by Henderson and associates (1994). These investigators, recording from the inferior colliculus in animals after noise damage, showed an increased amplitude of the near field evoked potential one day to one month after exposure. This rather curious finding led to a number of theories of plasticity related to rapid neural reorganization. One theory is that neuronal tracts are already in place but simply are not expressed until there is damage to the system. This report has also led to some new thoughts about recruitment. The increased response seen by Henderson and colleagues after cochlear damage could easily be thought of as a physiologic basis of recruitment.

One of the most significant advances in auditory deprivation and plasticity has been shown in auditory cortex reorganization after peripheral hearing loss. Robertson and Irvine (1989) reported that the auditory cortex in guinea pigs undergoes alteration of tonotopicity secondary to partial cochlear hearing loss. More specifically, the cochlear representation in the auditory cortex changed its frequency to the lower adjacent frequencies that are intact in the cochlea. Similar results were found by Harrison and colleagues (1991) with kittens and by Schwaber and colleagues (1993) with monkeys. It appears that the auditory cortex will reorganize its tonotopic arrangement to match the frequencies that are intact in the cochlea so that the neural tissue remains viable. Hence, rather than not obtaining sufficient stimulation due to a damaged end organ, the cortex will shift its response to frequencies that are intact. In these animals, this process of cortical reorganization seems to take place in about two to three months (Robertson & Irvine, 1989; Schwaber et al., 1993).

Auditory deprivation in humans usually occurs as a result of hearing loss. Obviously, there are many contaminating factors that influence the study of deprivation and its effects on humans. Nonetheless, there are some interesting examples of auditory deprivation effects in the human species. Otitis media and its related hearing loss has been shown to have an influence on the auditory brain stem response (ABR) in children who have had chronic problems with this disorder. The ABR studies seem to be consistent, showing mild central auditory dysfunction (i.e., extended latencies of the later waves) (Folsom et al., 1983; Lenhardt et al., 1985; Gunnerson & Finitzo, 1991). Conductive hearing loss has also been shown to enhance temporary threshold shift (Katz, 1965) and have relatively long-term effects on speech perception (Brown, 1994).

Another audiologic measure, masking level differences (MLDs), has been shown to be smaller in children with strong histories of otitis than in normal control subjects (Pillsbury et al., 1991; Hall & Grose, 1993). However, after corrective surgery (myringotomy and tubes), the MLDs return to normal in one to three months (Hall & Grose, 1994). The significance of these studies is that masking level differences are mediated at the low auditory brain stem and thus are related to central auditory function. Moreover, these MLD studies show that mild deprivation (such as often caused by otitis media) appears to result in subtle central dysfunction, which can be reversed by reestablishing normal hearing sensitivity.

Speech perception also appears to be influenced by auditory deprivation. In a study of identical twins, one with a chronic history of otitis media the other with essentially no history of the disease, both were evaluated at 4 years of age with the Pediatric Speech Intelligibility Test. The twin with the history of otitis scored considerably lower than the twin who did not have this conductive problem (Brown, 1994). Another manner in which speech recognition has been shown to be affected by auditory deprivation is in people with hearing loss who wear hearing aids. A number of reports have shown that individuals who have had binaural hearing loss for a period of time, and wear one hearing aid, have higher scores in the aided ear as compared to the unaided ear. In fact, the nonaided ear, over a period of time, in some cases showed a steady degradation in speech recognition performance. Also, people who have worn only one hearing aid for several years and then obtain a second device show an increase in speech recognition scores for the ear with the second aid (see Hurley, 1993; Silman et al., 1984). In other words, some reports have shown that a reversible effect can occur subsequent to supplying the "deprived" ear with more acoustic stimulation. Hence, in this clinically relevant example, there appears to be evidence of potential deprivation as well as an effect of stimulation on the auditory system. Auditory plasticity may be expressed by deprivation as well as stimulation effects, and it is the stimulation effect that is presented next.

Auditory Stimulation

Appropriate auditory stimulation can result in changes in the neural auditory system. This has been postulated for many years but experimental evidence has been slow to confirm it. However, some recent studies have provided some fascinating data. One of the earlier studies showed that white rats raised in an environment that provided a varied and systematic sound stimulation had auditory corticies that were different from those of control animals that were raised in normal sound environments (Hassmannova et al., 1981). The animals that were stimulated acoustically showed (near field) cortical potentials that were of shorter latency, and there were greater RNA concentrations in the auditory cortex, compared to matched controls (see Figure 2.1). This early study demonstrated that acoustic stimulation apparently influenced both functional and structural changes of the auditory cortex in animals.

FIGURE 2.1   Mean Latencies of Near Field (Auditory Cortex) Auditory Evoked Potentials from a Control and Experimental Group of Animals. The control group was raised in a "normal" environment, and the experimental group experienced several weeks of systematic acoustic stimulation.

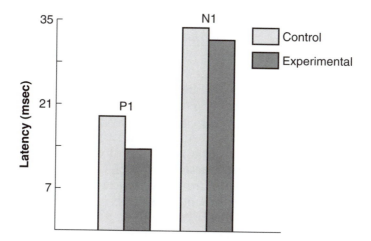

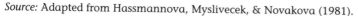

Source: Adapted from Hassmannova, Myslivecek, & Novakova (1981).

Knudsen (see Knudsen, 1988, for review) has reported evidence of similar plasticity in sound localization of barn owls. In this research, one ear was plugged on young barn owls and then localization errors were monitored. (These owls need acoustic feedback to fly to a designated target, hence their auditory systems are constantly activated and stimulated.) Initially, the barn owls' localization ability was hampered as expected, but after about two to three weeks, the owls' localization ability improved to near normal. After reaching near normal localization with one ear plugged, the plug was then removed. The localization became abnormal again but improved to normal in approximately one to two weeks. In other words, the neural substrate had adjusted to the different sound field cues caused by plugging one ear, and when the plug was removed, the neural substrate again changed to permit appropriate function. Knudsen also showed that auditory neurons in the barn owls changed their spatial tuning when the ear was plugged and unplugged, providing a physiological correlate to the behavioral localization changes and evidence of neural plasticity.

Another example of the effects of acoustic stimulation was a report by Recanzone and associates (1991). In this study, monkeys were trained on a frequency discrimination task within a small range of frequencies. Tonotopic mapping of the auditory cortex was performed after frequency discrimination training and compared to a control group of animals. The trained group of animals showed from two to eight times larger area of the frequency region used in training. The difference limen for frequency in the experimental group of monkeys improved over several weeks of training. This behavioral improvement was consistent with the anatomical changes noted in the auditory cortex. Changes in tuning of auditory cortex neurons was also noted in a study where guinea pigs were trained on a frequency discrimination task (Edeline & Weinberger, 1993).

The kinds of studies just mentioned have motivated researchers to employ auditory training with children who suffer from various auditory/language learning problems. This thinking, not really different from what happened in AT many years ago, was given a "new look" due to the impressive scientific data that surfaced. Most notable are the studies by Merzenich and associates (1996) and Tallal and associates (1996). These two studies show improvement in children with language learning problems with auditory temporal training and training on time extended and amplified transitions of speech. These well-controlled studies show the importance of AT and demonstrate how AT can improve performance. These are factors critical to the acceptance of AT as a clinical entity.

APPLICATIONS OF AUDITORY TRAINING/STIMULATION

Clinical Populations

Auditory training methodologies can be employed with various types of auditory processing problems; however, individuals with some types of CAPD may profit more than others. Since AT is dependent on brain plasticity to a great degree, the younger the patient, the better. Children with CAPD who have a neuromaturational lag certainly are among the prime candidates for intense AT. As mentioned earlier, maturation is dependent on stimulation, and AT may well serve as stimulation to the auditory system. An immature auditory system may lag in attaining some of its complex function but it also may have greater plasticity than more mature systems. It must be remembered that plasticity, maturation, and stimulation are all related (Kalil, 1989) (see Figure 2.2).

Auditory training can and should play a major role in neurological disorders. Stroke patients—especially those with characteristics of receptive aphasia—can profit from AT. The development of auditory skills that have been lost secondary to brain damage is dependent on stimulation and tasks that challenge the auditory system. However, even in cases of neurological damage, age becomes a factor, as younger people recover more quickly than do older people. A bigger issue, however, is that in cases of receptive aphasia, appropriate, systematic AT is necessary to best help the patient, and in many clinical situations this kind of therapy is not performed.

General Principles in Auditory Training

The recent research related to auditory plasticity, stimulation, and deprivation (depicted earlier) can illustrate some key concepts in AT. The

FIGURE 2.2 Relationships between Maturation, Stimulation, and Plasticity

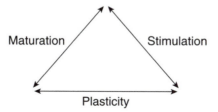

first concept of AT is that the brain (CANS and related systems) has the quality of plasticity and can be altered by acoustic stimulation or lack of it. The types of neural changes that are noted are neurochemical, physiological, and structural. It is reasonable to assume that appropriate AT can result in neural changes that will enhance auditory performance. Certainly behavioral and physiological evidence now exists to show that auditory stimulation/training does have an effect on audition.

Another concept key to AT is that brain plasticity is inversely related to brain maturation. The use and success of AT is related to plasticity, hence the younger the patient, the better the final results. Kalil's (1989) work has clearly shown that stimulation of neural tissue influences its maturation. The shaping of changes in the CANS can be accomplished better in a younger system. It must be remembered, however, that plasticity is still present in the mature system, and one should not think that AT will not be of value to the mature individual.

A third concept of AT is that the degree of neuronal change and growth is dependent on the type of stimulation and the task at hand. The clinical implication to this is that the type of training needs to be varied. A wide variety of auditory tasks and stimuli will generally be of greater value than those that are narrow in focus. However, this training should be directed by the results of previous tests and the history of the patient. In some cases, a narrow-focused therapy may be best if the deficit is very specific and well defined—often this is not the case, however. Task difficulty must be carefully monitored so that it is challenging but not overwhelming. Tasks that are too difficult do not help the system and they kill the patient's motivation. We like to use a 30-70 rule—at least 30 percent but not more than 70 percent success rate. The auditory tasks/stimuli should be presented systematically and be progressive in their complexity. Most indications also support the notion that AT must be intensive in regard to the content of the session and the number of sessions over time (Tallal et al., 1996).

OVERVIEW OF AUDITORY TRAINING TECHNIQUES

It is beyond the scope of this chapter to detail AT programs with which we have worked. However, we would like to provide an annotated outline of our "catalogue" of AT exercises. This may provide insight as to what we attempt to do in our clinic in regard to this one aspect (AT) for management of CAPD. We will use the categorization mentioned earlier: analytic, synthetic, pragmatic, and eclectic.

Analytic: Nonspeech

Some exercises in this category include intensity, frequency, and duration discrimination tasks. Also, the discrimination of intensity and frequency transitions can be useful. This requires the patient to determine the direction of change: up versus down for frequency; loud versus soft for intensity. We also employ a task where the frequency change and the speed of a "warble tone" can be varied. This provides practice for temporal and frequency discrimination. Training on temporal processes may include gap-detection tasks, sequencing tasks (two or more acoustic elements with the interstimulus interval and element duration adapted), and temporal discrimination tasks. Also, the detection and discrimination of rhythmic sequences can be included.

Localization of target stimuli (speech or nonspeech) with competing noise or multispeaker babble can help train subtle processes needed in everyday complex listening environments. This is set up in a traditional sound room (with noise in one speaker and speech in the other), with the subject changing positions to provide differing signal-to-noise ratios at each ear, as well as changing localization cues.

Analytic: Speech

Vowel, consonant, and blend identification and discrimination tasks can be attacked in a variety of ways. Sloan (1986) provides some excellent materials for training on these kinds of tasks. Discrimination of rhyme or words that are similar sounding provides an exercise that is highly relevant to many troubling listening situations. Temporal ordering of consonant-vowels or single consonants and vowels while varying the interstimulus interval is another task oriented toward those with temporal processing difficulties (see Merzenich et al., 1996). Listening to and identifying the prosodic elements in speech (in single words and in running speech) can also provide a challenge to temporal abilities.

Synthetic: Speech

The synthetic method of AT requires the use of contextual information. Training on the understanding of low-redundancy speech messages to improve auditory closure is a possibility. Auditory monitoring and feedback can be accomplished by reading aloud and checking comprehension. The naming of objects with only tactile cues (feeling the object) and or dichotic listening with varied intensity differences between channels (ears) can provide for interhemispheric stimulation.

Pragmatic: Speech and Nonspeech

Pragmatic AT is when the listener controls (or has controlled for them) acoustical factors such as intensity, signal-to-noise ratio, and so on. Tallal and associates' (1996) recent work of time expansion and intensity enhancement of speech transitions fits this category and obviously deserves consideration as a therapy technique. Auditory training using assistive listening devices that can help in recognizing subtle acoustic elements critical to speech identification can be a useful exercise. We have found this to be the case especially in learning to identify and discriminate vowels. There are also electronic devices in experimental stages that reportedly slow down speech without distortion. These kinds of devices would have strong AT implications for individuals with various types of temporal processing problems.

Deciding which of these exercises should be used has to be determined by testing as well as the educational, communicative, and medical history of the patient. In some cases, only one or two activities may be appropriate; in other cases, possibly none would be appropriate. Remember, AT is only one aspect of the total management approach to CAPD. In some instances, maximal use of strategies in listening and learning, overall education, and awareness may be the key to helping those with CAPD.

SUMMARY

This chapter related some aspects of CANS function to auditory training. It seems clear that improvement in auditory function and overall communication related to AT is secondary to changes in the CANS. These changes can be brought about by stimulation and training of the auditory system. Plasticity is a key property of the CANS that permits change in function and structure to evolve. Concepts of LTP, auditory deprivation, and brain changes related to auditory stimulation are all aspects of brain plasticity. The challenge in present-day audiology is to design AT programs that can make maximum use of brain plasticity to enhance one's auditory perception and overall communication. Some of the historic AT procedures may help professionals in this quest, but the time is right for new and innovative techniques of AT that take into account important neuroauditory concepts of hearing and hearing disorders.

REFERENCES

Alexander, D., & Frost, B. (1982). Decelerated synthesized speech as a means of shaping speech of auditory processing of children with delayed language. *Perception and Motor Skills, 5,* 783–792.

Bailey, C. H., & Chen, M. (1988). Long-term memory in *Aplysia* modulates the total number of varicosities of single indentified sensory neurons. *Proclamations of the National Academy of Sciences of the U.S.A., 85,* 2373–2377.

Blamey, P., & Alcantara, J. (1994). Research in auditory training. In J. Gagne & N. Tye-Murray (Eds.), Research in audiological rehabilitation [Monograph]. *J. Acad. Rehab. Audiology, 27,* 161–192.

Bliss, T. V. P., & Gardner-Medwin, A. R. (1973). Long-lasting potentiation of synaptic transmission in the dentate area of the unanaesthetized rabbit following stimulation of the perforant path. *Journal of Physiology, 232,* 357–374.

Bliss, T. V. P., & Lomo, T. (1973). Long-lasting potentiation of synaptic transmission in the dentate area of the anaesthetized rabbit following stimulation of the perforant path. *Journal of Physiology, 232,* 331–356.

Brown, D. P. (1994). Speech recognition in recurrent otitis media: Results in a set of identical twins. *Journal of the American Academy of Audiology, 5*(1), 1–6.

Carhart, R. (1960). Auditory training. In H. Davis (Ed.), *Hearing and deafness.* New York: Holt, Rinehart and Winston.

Chermak, G., & Musiek, F. (1992). Managing central auditory processing disorders in children and youth. *American Journal of Audiology, 1,* 62–65.

Chermak, G., & Musiek, F. (1997). *Central auditory processing disorders: New perspectives.* San Diego: Singular Press.

Clopton, B., & Silverman, N. (1978). Changes in latency and duration of a neural response following developmental auditory deprivation. *Experimental Brain Research, 32,* 39–47.

DiCarlo, L. M. (1948). Auditory training for the adult. *Volta Review, 50,* 490.

Doehring, D., & Ling, D. (1971). Programmed instruction of hearing impaired children in the auditory discrimination of vowels. *Journal of Speech and Hearing Research, 14,* 746.

Edeline, J. M., & Weinberger, N. M. (1993). Receptive field plasticity in the auditory cortex during frequency discrimination training: Selective retuning independent of task difficulty. *Behavioral Neuroscience, 107*(1), 82–103.

Erber, N. (1982). Auditory training. Washington DC: Alexander Graham Bell Association for the Deaf.

Evans, W., Webster, D., & Cullen, J. (1983). Auditory brainstem responses in neonatally sound deprived CBA/J mice. *Hearing Research, 10,* 269–277.

Folsom, R., Weber, B., & Thompson, G. (1983). Auditory brainstem responses in children with early recurrent middle ear disease. *Annals of Otology, Rhinology & Laryngology, 92,* 249–253.

Gengel, R., & Hirsh, I. (1970). Temporal order: The effect of single versus repeated presentations, practice, and verbal feedback. *Perception and Psychophysics, 7,* 209–216.

Greenough, W. T., & Bailey, C. H. (1988). The anatomy of a memory: Convergence of results across a diversity of tests. *Trends in Neuroscience, 11,* 142–146.

Gunnerson, A., & Finitzo, T. (1991). Conductive hearing loss during infancy: Effects on later auditory brainstem electrophysiology. *Journal of Speech and Hearing Research, 34,* 1207–1215.

Hall, J. G. (1976). The cochlear nuclei in monkeys after dihydrostreptomycin or noise exposure. *Acta Otolaryngologica, 81,* 344–352.

Hall, J., & Grose, J. (1993). The effect of otitis media with effusion on the masking level difference and the auditory brainstem response. *Journal of Speech & Hearing Research, 36,* 210–216.

Hall, J., & Grose, J. (1994). Development of temporal resolution in children as measured by the temporal modulation transfer function. *Journal of the Acoustical Society of America, 96,* 150–154.

Harrison, R. V., Nagasawa, A., Smith, D. W., Stanton, S., & Mount, R. J. (1991). Reorganization of auditory cortex after neonatal high frequency cochlear hearing loss. *Hearing Research, 54,* 11–19.

Hassmannova, J., Myslivecek, J., & Novakova, V. (1981). Effects of early auditory stimulation on cortical centers. In J. Syka & L. Aitkin (Eds.), *Neuronal mechanisms of hearing* (pp. 355–359). New York: Plenum.

Hebb, D. O. (1949). *The organization of behavior.* New York: John Wiley & Sons.

Henderson, D., Salvi, R., Boettcher, F., & Clock, A. (1994). Neurophysiologic correlates of sensorineural hearing loss. In J. Katz (Ed.), *Handbook of clinical audiology* (pp. 37–55). Baltimore: Williams & Wilkins.

Hudgins, C. V. (1954). Auditory training: Its possibilities and limitations. *Volta Review, 56,* 339.

Huizing, H. C. (1952). Auditory training. *Acta Otolaryngologica, 100* (Suppl.), 158.

Hurley, R. (1993). Monaural hearing aid effect: Case presentations. *Journal of the American Academy of Audiology, 4,* 285–295.

Kalil, R. (1989). Synapse formation in the developing brain. *Scientific American, 261,* 76–87.

Katz, J. (1965). Temporary threshold shift, auditory sensory deprivation, and conductive hearing loss. *Journal of the Acoustical Society of America, 37,* 923–924.

Katz, J. (1983). Phonemic synthesis. In E. Lasky & J. Katz (Eds.), *Central auditory processing disorders: Problems of speech language and learning* (pp. 269–296). Baltimore: University Park Press.

Katz, J., & Harmon, C. (1982). *Phonemic synthesis: Blending sounds into words.* Allan, TX: Developmental Learning Materials.

Kelly, J. C. (1954). A summer residential program in hearing education. *Journal of Speech and Hearing Disorders, 19,* 17.

Knudsen, E. (1988). Experience shapes sound localization and auditory unit properties during development in the barn owl. In G. Edelman, W. Gall, & W. Kowen (Eds.), *Auditory function: Neurobiological basis of hearing* (pp. 137–152). New York: John Wiley & Sons.

Lenhardt, M., Shaia, F., & Abedi, E. (1985). Brainstem evoked responses: Waveform variation associated with recurrent otitis media. *Archives of Otolaryngology, 111,* 315–316.

Lund, R. (1978). *Development and plasticity of the brain: An introduction*. New York: Oxford University Press.

Merzenich, M. M., Jenkins, W. M., Johnston, P., Schreiner, C., Miller, S. L., & Tallal, P. (1996). Temporal processing deficits of language-learning impaired children ameliorated by training. *Science, 271*, 77–80.

Morest, K. (1983). Degeneration of the brain following exposure to noise. In R. Hamernik, D. Henderson, & R. Salvi (Eds.), *New perspectives on noise induced hearing loss* (pp. 87–94). New York: Raven Press.

Musiek, F., & Chermak, G. (1995). Three commonly asked questions about central auditory processing disorders: Management. *American Journal of Audiology, 4*, 15–18.

Neisser, V., & Hirst, W. (1974). Effect of practice on the identification of auditory sequences. *Perception and Psychophysics, 15*, 391–395.

Pierson, M., & Synder-Keller, A. (1994). Development of frequency-selective domains in inferior colliculus of normal and neonatally noise-exposed rats. *Brain Research, 636*(1), 55–67.

Pillsbury, H., Grose, J., & Hall, J. (1991). Otitis media with effusion in children. *Arch. Otolaryngol., Head and Neck Surg., 117*, 718–723.

Recanzone, G., Schreiner, C., Hradek, G., Sutter, M., Beitel, R., & Merzenich, M. (1991). Functional reorganization of the primary auditory cortex in adult own monkeys parallel improvements in performance in an auditory frequency discrimination task. *Society for Neuroscience Abstracts, 17*, 534.

Robertson, D., & Irvine, D. R. F. (1989). Plasticity of frequency organization in auditory cortex of guinea pigs with partial unilateral deafness. *Journal of Comparative Neurology, 282*, 456–471.

Rogan, M. T., & LeDoux, J. E. (1995). LTP is accompanied by commensurate enhancement of auditory-evoked responses in a fear conditioning circuit. *Neuron, 15*(1), 127–136.

Rosenzweig, M. R., Bennett, E. L., & Krech, D. (1964). Cerebral effects of environmental complexity and training among adult rats. *Journal of Comparative and Physiological Psychology, 57*(3), 438–439.

Sanders, D. A. (1971). *Aural rehabilitation*. Englewood Cliffs, NJ: Prentice Hall.

Scheich, H. (1991). Auditory cortex: Comparative aspects of maps and plasticity. *Current Opinion in Neurobiology, 1*, 236–247.

Schow, R., & Nerbonne, M. (1996). *Introduction to audiologic rehabilitation* (3rd ed., pp. 81–117). Boston: Allyn and Bacon.

Schwaber, M., Garraghty, P., & Kaas, J. (1993). Neuroplasticity of the adult primate auditory cortex. *Am. J. Otology, 14*, 252–258.

Silman, S., Gelfand, S., & Silverman, C. (1984). Late onset auditory deprivation: Effects of monaural versus binaural hearing aids. *Journal of the Acoustical Society of America, 76*, 1357–1362.

Sloan, C. (1986). *Treating auditory processing difficulties in children*. San Diego: College-Hill Press.

Stout, G., & Windle, J. (1992). *Developmental approach to successfull listening II*. Engelwood, CO: Resource Point.

Tallal, P., Miller, S. L., Bedi, G., Byma, G., Wang, X., Nagarajan, S. S., Schreiner, C., Jenkins, W. M., & Merzenich, M. M. (1996). Language comprehension in language-learning impaired children improved with acoustically modified speech. *Science, 271,* 81–84.

Tucci, D., Born, D., & Rubel, E. (1987). Changes in spontaneous activity in CNS morphology associated with conductive and sensorineural hearing loss in chickens. *Annals of Otology, Rhinology and Laryngology, 96,* 343–350.

Walden, B., Erdman, I., Montgomery, A., Schwartz, D., & Prosek, R. (1981). Some effects of training on speech recognition by hearing impaired adults. *Journal of Speech & Hearing Research, 24,* 207–216.

Walgar, M., Laska, M., Schneider, I., Diekmann, H., & von Wedel, H. (1993). Maturation of auditory evoked potentials in young guinea pigs with binaural conductive hearing loss. *European Archives of Otorhinolaryngology, 250*(6), 362–365.

Webster, D. (1983). A critical period during postnatal auditory development in mice. *International Journal of Pediatric Otorhinolaryngology, 6,* 107–118.

Webster, D. (1988). Sound amplification negates central effects of neonatal conductive hearing loss. *Hearing Research, 32,* 192–195.

Webster, D., & Webster, M. (1977). Neonatal sound deprivation affects brainstem auditory nuclei. *Archives of Otolaryngology, 103,* 392–396.

Wedenberg, E. (1951). Auditory training of the deaf and hard of hearing children. *Acta Otolaryngologica, 94* (Suppl.), 1–129.

3

THE RELATIONSHIP BETWEEN ATTENTION DEFICIT HYPERACTIVITY DISORDER, CENTRAL AUDITORY PROCESSING DISORDERS, AND SPECIFIC LEARNING DISORDERS

WARREN D. KELLER
Private Practice, East Amherst, New York

One Saturday morning not long ago, I was waiting in line at our local bagel shop when a colleague of mine, a school psychologist, approached me to discuss a youngster who he had just evaluated and who had been referred to me for further neuropsychological evaluation. This was an extremely bright, competent child whose measured intelligence fell within the very superior range, based on standardized intellectual tests. Although he was not yet 11 years old, the child had a history of psychiatric hospitalization and was struggling both at home and at school. This was in part due to clear obsessive-compulsive features to his behavioral and emotional functioning. Although I had not yet evaluated the child, the school psychologist wanted me to know that "the kid is fine. . . . After all, his IQ is 135!"

In recalling some of the information that I had reviewed for this child, I remembered that he had been evaluated by Dr. Katz and was found to have evidence of a central auditory processing (CAP) dysfunction with a tolerance-fading memory profile. When I mentioned this to my school psychologist colleague, he responded, "We have a big problem with Dr. Katz." My first thought was, How in the world could anyone have a problem with Jack Katz? My colleague elaborated, "We don't trust him; he sees something wrong with everyone." Again, I found it hard to understand how there could continue to be a negative reaction on the part of so many individuals to the notion that an individual might have CAPDs and that that how one processes auditory information might not have an impact on one's academic and behavioral functioning. Taking a neuropsychological perspective, we know that the "brain pumps behavior" just like the "heart pumps blood," and deviations in auditory processing behavior, just as deviations in any other type of behavior, might well have implications for brain organization and development.

I believe that one of the reasons for my colleague's suspiciousness is the lack of understanding of the true nature and implications of CAP disorders. Furthermore, the lack of predictive validity leads certain individuals to be more suspicious of the notion of CAP dysfunction. Lastly, we all approach the understanding of a child from our own professional disciplines and personal biases. This single-discipline approach, as opposed to a transdisciplinary approach, will serve only to inhibit our understanding of development, learning, and learning disorders.

THE RELATIONSHIP BETWEEN CAPDs AND ADHD

The relationship between auditory skills, language, and attention seems to be an intimate one. Baker and Cantwell (1987) have demonstrated that preschoolers with speech and language delays are more likely to be diagnosed as having an attention deficit hyperactivity disorder (ADHD) as well. Children with ADHD, a neurobiological disorder, experience difficulties with sustained attention; they are impulsive and highly distractible. Although many children with ADHD experience coexisting learning disorders, the majority of these children experience problems with significant underachievement in school settings.

This close relationship between language disturbances during the preschool years and difficulties with sustained attention, impulsivity, and distractibility has been supported by others (Love & Thompson, 1988). It has been proposed that CAPDs and ADHD may even reflect a singular disorder (Gascon, Johnson, & Burd, 1986), since children with evidence of central auditory processing dysfunction showed an improvement on CAP tests when they were provided stimulant medication. The similarities in children with both ADHD and CAPDs can be appreciated by reviewing the characteristics of these children described in Figure 3.1. Children who experience an auditory perceptual disorder present with difficulties very similar to children with an attention deficit disorder. In addition, children who are inattentive, impulsive, and highly distractible may clearly present as if they had specific auditory processing disorders. My impression, based on both my clinical work with children and my reading of the limited but growing literature in this area, is that ADHD and CAPDs are not a singular developmental disorder. Rather, CAPDs are likely separate disorders from ADHD. Both CAPDs and ADHD may occur independently or in conjunction with each other.

Children presenting with attentional difficulties represent a very heterogenous group. Difficulties with sustained attention may be due to auditory perceptual dysfunctions, an attention deficit hyperactivity disorder, childhood depression, childhood anxiety, oppositional defiant disorder, learning disabilities, a chaotic disorganized family situation, or situational stresses that might be reflective of some trauma that the child has experienced. A very comprehensive, differential diagnosis must be made of an attention deficit disorder. Much of the research investigating the relationship between CAPDs and ADHD has identified children with ADHD based on either physician report or standardized behavioral questionnaires. This method of identifying children with ADHD provides little assurance that the children selected for study truly have ADHD. The limitations of the use of only standardized questionnaires and physician reports in diagnosing ADHD have been thoroughly discussed elsewhere (Goldstein & Goldstein, 1989; Gordon, 1991).

Burd and Fisher (1986) have argued that CAP tests do not provide an adequate measure of auditory processing capabilities, since they appear to measure little else other than attention. They questioned whether APD existed independent of ADHD. Gascon, Johnson, and Burd (1986) found that in a relatively small sample of 19 children with ADHD, 79 percent of these children evidenced CAPDs, suggesting a close degree of overlap between ADHD and CAPDs. Some 86 percent of these children improved their performance on CAP tests when provided stimulant medication in a double-blind, placebo-controlled, single-crossover study of methylphenidate. Also, 80 percent of the subjects with ADHD also met the criteria for CAPDs, again indicating the close overlap between these two disorders.

A significant difference was found on some of the dependent variables when comparing medicated versus nonmedicated conditions, but other variables—such as responses on the Staggered Spondaic Word (SSW) Test—were dropped from further analysis, presumably because there were no differences. The authors concluded that sustained atten-

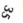
Characteristics of Children with ADHD and CAPD

Deficit Hyperactivity Disorder (ADHD)

General Characteristics
Inability to sustain attention
  Impaired focused attention
  Impaired selective attention
  Impaired divided attention
  Impaired vigilance

Symptoms Often Seen in School Setting
Disorganization
Short attention span
Impulsivity
Problems completing work
  Work completed impulsively
  Takes too long to complete work
Chronic academic underachievement
Variability in academic performance
Messy work, often carelessly done
Failure to follow instructions
Motor restlessness
Noisy/excessive talking

Associated Features
Cognitive deficits
  Specific learning disabilities
  Auditory processing disorders
  Problems with visual perceptual
    processing
  Academic underachievement for
    intelligence

Central Auditory Processing Disorder (CAPDs)

General Characteristics
Says "huh" or "what" frequently
Gives inconsistent responses to
  auditory stimuli
Often misunderstands what is said
Constantly requests that information
  be repeated
Has poor auditory attention
Is easily distracted
Has difficulty following oral
  instructions
Has difficulty listening in the presence
  of background noise

Has difficulty with phonics and
  speech-sound discrimination
Has poor auditory memory (span and
  sequence)
Has poor receptive and expressive
  language
Gives slow or delayed response to
  verbal stimuli
Has reading, spelling, and other
  academic problems
Learns poorly through the auditory
  channel
Exhibits behavior problems

Emotional Difficulties
Temper tantrum/explosive behavior
Low self-esteem
Problems interpreting other's
  emotions
Low frustration tolerance
Mood swings
Hyperactivity/hyperemotionality

Social Difficulties
Poor peer relations
Problems with taking turns
Impulsiveness
Hyperactivity
Aggressiveness
Noncompliance
Lying/stealing
Poor self-control
Poor general social skills
Alcohol/drug abuse

Physical Features
Poor general health
Enuresis/encopresis
Increased incidence of otitis media
Increased frequency of allergies/food
  sensitivities
Greater frequency of disturbance in
  sleep/wake cycles
Poor motor coordination
Suspected underaroused central
  nervous system
Greater frequency of minor physical
  anomalies
Familial pattern to the disorder

tion was a critical feature of performance on CAPD tests. They suggested that the available diagnostic criteria for CAPDs might make a clinical separation of the two disorders problematic. They further suggested, rather prematurely, that stimulant medication appears to be a useful treatment for the symptoms of both ADHD and CAPDs.

Keith and Engineer (1991) found significant improvement in some auditory processing abilities, auditory vigilance tasks, and performance on the Token Test when children were receiving stimulant medication. The study indicated that performance on attention-dependent tasks may be improved when children with attentional difficulties are provided stimulant medication, but the study was not designed to address the issues surrounding comorbidity of these two disorders. It must be kept in mind that stimulant medication results in improvement of sustained attention in normal children as well as in children with ADHD.

Tillery (1992) found that 83 percent of a sample of children with ADHD also met the criteria for CAPDs, but she found little improvement on central auditory tasks when comparing medicated versus nonmedicated performance. Riccio, Hynd, Cohen, and Molt (1994) have more recently provided evidence that ADHD and CAPD are separate diagnostic entities. In a sample of 38 children demonstrating impairment on the SSW test, 55 percent also met the diagnostic criteria for ADHA. They found little correlation between SSW performance and teacher ratings on standardized questionnaires assessing ADHD symptomatology. They then argued that SSW performance was probably not reflective of problems with attention, impulsivity, and hyperactivity. It needs to be kept in mind, however, that these were reported behavioral features associated with ADHD as measured by these particular teacher report scales. More objective measures of vigilance may not have provided the same results.

Riccio and colleagues (1994) also investigated whether any specific pattern of impairment on the SSW test might be associated with the diagnosis of ADHD. Although they argued that there was no specific pattern of impairment on the SSW that was associated with those children in their sample who met their diagnostic criteria for ADHD, 52 percent of those children with ADHD fell into the tolerance-fading memory profile based on their performance on the SSW. Riccio and colleagues argued that their data supported the notion that performance on the SSW test and CAP disturbances could not be explained solely by disturbances in attention, impulsivity, and hyperactivity.

The one replicated finding from the preceding studies is that among a sample of children meeting the criteria for CAPD, there is a substantioal number who also meet the diagnostic criteria for ADHD. For the clinician, considerable effort needs to be placed into being able to consider when APD might really be ADD, when ADD might really be APD, and when APD and ADD might be coexisting. Clinicians need to be sensitive to the characteristics of both ADD and APD in order to ensure that the most appropriate management and treatment of their patients is provided (Keller, 1992).

THE RELATIONSHIP BETWEEN CAPD AND SPECIFIC LEARNING DISABILITIES

The relationship between ADHD and specific learning disorders is well documented. Generally, it is believed that 25 to 40 percent of children with ADHD will also experience a specific learning disability capable of adversely impacting their academic achievement (Barkley, 1990). Given the relationship between ADHD and specific learning disorders, and given the relationship between ADHD and CAPDs, it is not surprising that there would be a relationship between CAPDs and specific learning disorders.

In one sample of 94 children with learning disabilities, only 1 child was free from CAP dysfunction (Katz, 1992). Katz has described the specific types of learning deficits that characterize the various categories of performance on the SSW test. For example, the decoding category, characterized by a particular pattern of results on the SSW test, is associated with poor phonemic synthesis skills; delayed reading, spelling, and phonics; and weaknesses in both receptive language and articulation. In contrast, the tolerance-fading memory category, rather than being associated with some dysfunction in the left posterior temporal area, is postulated to be associated with weaknesses in the frontal area. In contrast to the poor phonemic skills characterizing those individuals in the decoding category, individuals who exhibit the tolerance-fading memory profile have been described as having well-developed decoding skills and spelling skills, but weaker reading comprehension, expressive language problems, and poor handwriting.

NEUROPSYCHOLOGICAL SUBTYPES OF CHILDREN WITH SPECIFIC LEARNING DISORDERS

It is well accepted that learning disabilities do not constitute a singular developmental disorder. Neuropsychologists have made significant progress since the 1960s in identifying specific subtypes of learning disabilities (Rourke, 1985). The factors preventing a child from learning to read are different from the factors preventing a child from learning to spell, from learning to make arithmetic calculations, and so on. All children with learning disabilities are not created equally and neither are all children with CAP disturbances. In order to effectively manage and remediate the deficits of children with specific learning disabilities, practitioners need to be able to describe and understand the specific deficiencies those children experience. Effective management strategies for the dyscalculic child will be very different from the management strategies most effective for the dyslexic child. Might the categories of CAP disturbances proposed by Katz be associated with specific subtypes of learning disorders proposed by others (Rourke, 1985)?

NONVERBAL LEARNING DISORDERS (NLD SYNDROME)

Rourke and colleagues (Rourke, 1985, 1989) have described a particular subtype of learning disability that they refer to as the *nonverbal learning disability (NLD)* syndrome after the seminal works of Helmer Myklebust (1975). Neuropsychological studies that have focused on the heterogeneity of children with learning disabilities have fostered a better, more comprehensive understanding of this particular syndrome of learning disorder. The primary neuropsychological deficits that these children experience include significant weaknesses in visuospatial functioning and graphomotor skills, with tactile-perceptual deficits often more marked on the left side of the body (Gross-Tsur, Shalev, Manor, & Amir, 1995).

Individuals with the NLD syndrome classically experience a great deal of difficulty when exposed to novel material and when they are asked to utilize problem-solving strategies in situations not previously experienced. Attentional weaknesses, especially to visual and tactile information, are typically pronounced. While the syndrome has been described as being "nonverbal" in nature, these individuals also evidence speech and language difficulties. Although they might be quite verbose, psycholinguistic pragmatics may be poor, and they may engage in what has been referred to as "cocktail party" speech. Speech prosody is also an area in which these individuals may show weaknesses. In contrast to these neuropsychological deficits, these children have clear strengths. Auditory perceptual capabilities may *appear* very well developed and phonetic analysis skills may be exceptionally strong.

Figure 3.2 provides some of the more salient characteristics of a nonverbal learning disorder. This particular subtype of learning disability clearly is a syndrome in that it has implications for early development, later development, intellectual functioning, academic functioning, as

FIGURE 3.2   Characteristics of Individuals with a Nonverbal Learning Disorder (NLD)

1. Developmental histories sometimes indicate precocious language development with slight delays in acquisition of motor milestones.
2. As infants, these children might have histories of tactile defensiveness, or at least were not thought of as cuddly.
3. As youngsters (below 8 years of age), these children are regarded as being immature.
4. As a group, these children are identified as learning disabled much later than usual. Boys tend to be identified somewhat earlier than girls, however.
5. These children are often regarded as clumsy or uncoordinated and as impulsive.
6. These children are usually thought of as being bright, but unmotivated and lazy.
7. These children are highly verbal and articulate. They will talk excessively in many situations, but express relatively little meaningful content (e.g., "cocktail party" speech).
8. Equal incidence occurs in males and females.
9. Generally, these children will interact well with adults, but exhibit poor social interactional skills with children (and may have few friends).
10. Intellectually, these children may have depressed performance scores, relative to verbal scores on the WISC-R.
11. Academically, these children have a characteristic profile of "hyperlexia" or at least average reading recognition skills. They may have a slow start in reading, exhibit poor reading comprehension, and have poor mechanical arithmetic abilities.
12. These children will exhibit a characteristic profile on personality evaluation. They will show peak scores on the Depression, Anxiety, Psychosis, and/or Withdrawal subscales of the Personality Inventory for Children. Often, they are referred for suspected primary emotional disturbance due to difficulties with their emotional functioning.
13. These children will show a characteristic pattern on neuropsychological evaluation:

    Sensory Impairments
    Bilateral Motor Impairments
      Fingertip Number Writing Recognition
      Finger Agnosia
      Suppressions on Double Simultaneous Stimulation
    Impairment of Category Test
    Depressed Scores on Tactual Performance Test, Target Test
    Dysgraphic Writing

well as socioemotional functioning. Often, the developmental presentation of this learning disorder may include the impression that the child is "hard of hearing" (Rourke, 1989) and that he or she may experience initial delays in the acquisition of speech. Most often, the syndrome is characterized by relative inactivity during infancy and toddlerhood.

Children appear much more sedentary than one might expect and they may evidence slight delays in acquisition of motor skills, with independent ambulation not occurring until 14 or 15 months of age. In one child, the parents reported enthusiasm at being able to continue dining at some of the finest French restaurants in the area while their 2-year-old would remain under the table, occupying himself throughout a leisurely dinner. These children develop fine phonemic hearing with good sound-blending skills and may be excessively verbal, talking in many situations. In contrast, they may present with gross deficiencies in the content and pragmatics of their speech. Since visuospatial functioning is a clear neuropsychological deficit, the academic presentation early on includes weaknesses in graphomotor skills and, typically, delays in acquisition of reading. Since visuospatial abilities are a clear prerequisite for reading acquisition, these children struggle with reading until later in development, perhaps the third grade or so, when their visual-perceptual abilities have matured to the point where they will support the acquisition of reading. At that time, word-decoding skills blossom and often will surpass their chronological age levels fairly quickly.

The child with NLD will usually exhibit pronounced weaknesses in graphomotor skills due to the bilateral motor impairments that typically characterize the syndrome. Oral spelling abilities may be quite strong, but their ability to write spelling words correctly may be the focus of some attention in school. When words are misspelled, they are typically phonetically quite accurate. Spelling skills are thought of as an academic asset, particularly beyond the fifth grade or so, when there tends to be an improvement in graphomotor abilities. Despite the difficulty with the early acquisition of reading, reading skills ultimately become an area of strength, with mechanical arithmetic abilities an area of pronounced deficit. Weaknesses in fine motor skills and spatial functioning often lead them to commit errors in "carrying," and arithmetic errors are also made due to their inability to keep numbers in columns easily.

Academically, organizational deficits and weaknesses in reading comprehension characterize the syndrome. On standardized testing, it would not be unusual for an adolescent with NLD to evidence reading recognition skills at a 12.9 grade level, computational arithmetic skills at a 5.6 grade level, spelling skills at an 11.0 grade level, with reading comprehension at a 7.0 grade level.

In addition to the predicted pattern of academic test scores, individuals exhibiting the NLD syndrome will typically obtain verbal scores on the Wechsler Scales significantly higher than performance scores on intellectual evaluation. There will most often be a statistically significant difference with higher verbal IQs, but in some cases, the difference will be more clinically significant than statistically.

Given the pattern of neuropsychological deficits that these individuals present with, it has been speculated that deficiencies in the right hemisphere may provide the neuroanatomical basis for the development of the syndrome. NLD syndrome is manifested in children who experience significant tissue removal from the right hemisphere. It also occurs more frequently in children who are survivors of acute lymphocytic leukemia, individuals who manifest dysgenesis of the corpus callosum, and hydrocephalic children, and it occurs more frequently in situations where there has been clear cerebral trauma. Features of the syndrome have also been described as being characteristic of individuals with pervasive developmental disorders and Asperger's syndrome.

Considerable research has demonstrated the contribution that the right hemisphere makes to emotional functioning. It is not surprising, then, that the NLD syndrome has implications with respect to behavioral and socioemotional functioning. Social problems tend to be a hallmark feature of the disorder. These children tend to experience far greater difficulty interpreting nonverbal social cues. Problem-solving skills, when language cues are removed, can be grossly impaired. Similarly, these children often experience difficulty expressing as well as understanding emotions. They may not be able to effectively interpret when someone is experiencing surprise, anger, or excitement, unless someone tells them. Social isolation is common. In severe cases, facial recognition skills may be impaired.

Individuals exhibiting NLD are believed to be at far greater risk for the development of internalizing symptomatology. Rates of depression, anxiety, and severe socioemotional disturbances are common among this group (Rourke, 1989; Strong & Rourke, 1985). On standardized measures of personality functioning, it is not unusual to see their parents report greater symptoms associated with depression, anxiety, withdrawal, and occasionally rather unusual, bizarre behavior. Rourke (1989) has suggested that individuals with this syndrome are at greater risk not only for depression but for suicide as well.

Given the attentional difficulties that these children present with, it is not unusual for them to be perceived as having ADHD at some point during their lives and to be tried on stimulant medication. Many of them will meet the diagnostic criteria for both NLD as well as ADHD (Strong & Rourke, 1985). Clinically, in my impression, they do not seem to respond as favorably to stimulant medications. Experts know that children who present with ADHD and experience the comorbid anxiety and depression that typically characterizes the NLD syndrome do not show as positive a response to stimulant medication and may well evidence greater side effects (Barkley, 1990).

In my work as a neuropsychologist assessing and treating children and adults with specific learning disorders, I have had the opportunity to work closely with audiologists over the past 20 years. Clinically, I observed children being diagnosed as having a tolerance-fading memory profile on central auditory processing evaluation often sharing many of the characteristics of children with either ADHD or the NLD syndrome. Children with NLD syndrome often will present similarly to children with ADHD and may meet diagnostic criteria for both disorders.

I believe there are some striking similarities between the descriptions of children evidencing a tolerance-fading memory profile on CAP testing to the descriptions of children with nonverbal learning disorders. The similarities between children with CAPDs and TFM profiles and children with NLD are evident in Table 3.1. Katz has described children with this auditory processing disability as also having the poor graphomotor skills, the poor reading comprehension, and the greater internalizing symptomatology that characterizes children with nonverbal learning disorders. It may well be that the SSW test is a valid method for discriminating individuals with particular subtypes of learning disability syndromes despite the label various professionals provide, given their different professional disciplines. The importance of subtype analysis is to be able to ultimately provide improved and more effective remediation strategies.

There are clear implications for remediation for individuals with NLD. For example, their learning tends to be more effective when a rote, repetitive approach to learning is employed. If it were demonstrated that a TFM profile on CAPD testing is, in fact, correlated with NLD syndrome, certainly my school psychologist colleague alluded to earlier in this chapter might not meet the diagnosis of CAPD with hesitancy and reluctance. I suspect that categories of central auditory processing dysfunction, such as the TFM profile, may be revealing far more about an individual than just how he or she processes auditory information. It is important to remember that this is, in fact, a tool that provides us with a "glimpse into the nervous system"—the same nervous system that "pumps behavior."

Riccio and colleagues (Riccio, Hynd, Cohen, & Molt, 1996) found that approximately 50 percent of children exhibiting a TFM profile on CAPD testing also met their diagnostic criteria for ADHD. Although they seemed to underestimate the importance of this finding, I am impressed with the fact that a particular profile on the SSW test is so closely associ-

TABLE 3.1 Relationships between Subtypes of Central Auditory Processing Disorders, Learning Disabilities, and Attention Deficit Disorder

Tolerance-Fading Memory	Attention Deficit Disorder (ADHD)	Nonverbal Learning Disorder (NLD)
Characteristics		
Poor auditory memory	Inattentive	Inattentive
Poor auditory figure-ground skills	Impulsive	Impulsive
Impulsive	Distractible	Distractible
Fearful		Greater degree of internalizing symptomatology
Insecure		Fearful
		Insecure
Neuroanatomical Weakness		
Anterior temporal	Frontal lobe functioning	Right hemisphere dysfunction
Frontal regions		Corpus callosal dysfunction
Academic Characteristics		
Distractible	Distractible	Distractible
Inconsistent articulation	Inconsistent articulation	Good articulation skills
Reading comprehension weak	Reading comprehension weak	Reading comprehension weaker than reading decoding
Good decoding skills	Variable decoding skills depending on associated learning problems	Good decoding skills
Weak expressive language	Weakness in motor skills often secondary to inattention	Weak expressive language (talks a lot but says little)
Poor motor programming and poor handwriting	Poor handwriting	Fine motor weaknesses in infancy and childhood, which often decrease with development
Difficulty following directions	Difficulty following directions	Poor handwriting
		Difficulty understanding directions
		Mathematics typically very weak

Incidence	Approximately 20% of population of LD children with CAPD	6 times greater in males (perhaps) 3 to 5% of population	Equal incidence in males and females Approximately 17% of LD population
Development	Unknown	70% of children with ADHD continue to evidence symptomotology into adulthood	Precocious language development not unusual with delayed aquisition of motor milestones NLD syndrome persists into adulthood
Intellectual Profile	Unknown	Variable	Suppressed performance scores on intellectual evaluation

ated with a subgroup of children whose difficulties might be diminished if they were prescribed stimulant medication. I would interpret their research findings as suggesting that children exhibiting TFM profiles on CAPD testing might be further evaluated for the presence of ADHD. Similarly, it may be that children exhibiting TFM profiles on CAPD testing may be highly correlated with the presence of an NLD syndrome. If this is the case, then the results of the auditory processing evaluation could actually be helpful in discriminating a group of children who are at great risk for severe internalizing symptoms and significant depression.

Researchers need to further explore the relationship between auditory processing capabilities and how they relate to other particular subtypes of learning disorders. Until these relationships are better understood, caution must be used. I had the occasion to review an audiological evaluation of a youngster diagnosed as having a TFM profile where it was recommended that this child utilize his better visual skills to help him compensate for his weaker auditory abilities. In this case, the TFM profile was, in fact, associated with a child exhibiting the NLD syndrome whose visuospatial abilities were far more deficient than his auditory and language abilities. It might well be a mistake to assume that since a youngster performs poorly on central auditory processing evaluation, his or her visual skills might be an area of strength. The possibility exists, in my estimation, that a TFM profile on CAPD testing may be helpful in discriminating children with impaired visuospatial abilities!

Research has clearly demonstrated the need for increased collaboration among professionals who work with children who have learning and attentional problems. Continued transdisciplinary research is required in order to obtain a more accurate, valid way of understanding when a youngster's learning and attentional difficulties may be due to CAPD, ADHD, and/or LD. Continuing to see developmental problems from a single professional discipline approach will inhibit one's ability to understand and develop effective management strategies. Effective diagnosis remains the most important prerequisite to effective management.

REFERENCES

Baker, L., & Cantwell, D. P. (1987). A prospective psychiatric follow-up of children with speech/language disorders. *Journal of the American Academy of Child Psychiatry, 26,* 546–553.

Barkley, R. (1990). *Attention deficit hyperactivity disorder: A handbook for diagnosis and treatment.* New York: Guilford Press.

Burd, L., & Fisher, W. (1986). Central auditory processing disorder or attention deficit disorder? *Dev. Behav. Pediatr., 7,* 215.

Cook, J. R., Mausbach, T., Burd, L., Gascon, G. G., Slotnick, H., Patterson, B., Johnson, R., Hankey, B., & Reynolds, B. (1993). A preliminary study of the relationship between central auditory processing and attention deficit disorder. *Journal of Psychiatry Neuroscience, 18*(3), 130–137.

Gascon, G. G., Johnson, R., & Burd, L. (1986). Central auditory processing and attention deficit disorders. *Journal of the Child Neurology, 1,* 27–33.

Goldstein, S., & Goldstein, M. (1989). *Managing attention disorders in children: A guide for practitioners.* New York: Wiley.

Gordon, M. (1991). *ADHD/Hyperactivity: A consumer's guide.* DeWitt, NY: GSI Publications.

Gross-Tsur, V., Shalev, R. S., Manor, O., & Amir, N. (1995). Developmental right-hemisphere syndrome: Clinical spectrum of the nonverbal learning disability. *Journal of the Learning Disabilities,* 80–86.

Katz, J. (1992). Classification of auditory processing disorders. In J. Katz, N. Stecker, & D. Henderson (Eds.), *Central auditory processing: A transdisciplinary view.* Chicago: Mosby.

Keith, R. W., & Engineer, P. (1991). Effects of methylphenidate on the auditory processing abilities of children with ADHD. *Journal of Learning Disabilities,* 630–636.

Keller, W. D. (1992). Auditory processing disorder or attention deficit disorder. In J. Katz, N. Stecker, & D. Henderson (Eds.), *Central auditory processing: A transdisciplinary view.* Chicago: Mosby.

Love, A. J., & Thompson, N. G. G. (1988). Language disorders and attention deficit disorders in young children referred for psychiatric services: Analysis of picualence and a conceptual synthesis. *American Journal of Orthopsychiatry, 58,* 52–64.

Myklebust, H. R. (1975). Nonverbal learning disabilities: Assessment and intervention. In H. R. Myklebust (Ed.), *Progress in learning disabilities* (pp. 85–121). New York: Grune and Stratton.

Riccio, C., Hynd, G. W., Cohen, M. J., Hall, J., & Molt, L. (1994). Comorbidity of central auditory processing disorder and attention deficit hyperactivity disorder. *Journal of the Academy at Child and Adolescent Psychiatry,* 849–857.

Riccio, C., Hynd, G. W., Cohen, M. J., & Molt, L. (1996). The staggered spondaic word test: Performance of children with attention-deficit hyperactivity disorder. *American Journal of Audiology, 5,* 55–62.

Rourke, B. P. (Ed.). (1985). *Neuropsychology of learning disabilities: Essentials of subtype analysis.* New York: Guilford Press.

Rourke, B. P. (Ed.). (1989). *Nonverbal learning disabilities: The syndrome and the model.* New York: Guilford Press.

Strong, J. D., & Rourke, B. P. (1985). Adaptive behavior of children with specific arithmetic disabilities and associated neuropsychological abilities and deficits. In B. P. Rourke (Ed.), *Neuropsychology of learning disabilities: Essentials of subtype analysis* (pp. 302–328). New York: Guilford Press.

Tillery, K. L. (1992). *Central auditory processing abilities of attention deficit hyperactivity disordered children: With and without methylphenidate.* Unpublished master's thesis, Illinois State University.

4

METACOGNITIVE APPROACHES TO MANAGING CENTRAL AUDITORY PROCESSING DISORDERS

GAIL D. CHERMAK
Washington State University

Management of central auditory processing disorders requires a comprehensive approach, given the range of listening and learning deficits associated with this complex and heterogeneous group of disorders (Chermak & Musiek, 1992). Improving listening skills and spoken language comprehension—primary intervention goals—are achieved by training the listener to interact actively with the acoustic signal, deploying linguistic, cognitive, and metacognitive systems to reconstruct a spoken message.

Clearly, auditory processing deficits are primary in causing a central auditory processing disorder (CAPD); however, since listening takes place within the multiple contexts of the acoustic, phonetic, linguistic, and social domains, simultaneous and integrated orchestration of multiple knowledge bases and skills is required for spoken language comprehension. Weaknesses or inefficiencies in linguistic, cognitive, or metacognitive domains can exacerbate CAPD, compounding the adverse impact of the sensory processing deficit for listening, communication, and learning (ASHA, 1996). Conversely, augmenting the function of these multiple

The material appearing in this chapter is an abridged version of material originally appearing in Chermak, G. D., and Musiek, F. E. (1997). *Central auditory processing disorders: New perspectives.* San Diego: Singular Publishing Group. Used with permission.

systems and knowledge bases in the service of spoken language comprehension offers opportunities for remediation.

Although not directly targeting central auditory processes, remediation strategies incorporating metalinguistic and metacognitive knowledge and processes can benefit listening and spoken language understanding. Moreover, because many of these strategies can benefit reading as well as listening comprehension, they may also reduce learning problems. For example, training in deducing word meaning from context should benefit both listening and reading comprehension, given the robust correlations among vocabulary, reading comprehension, and listening comprehension (Perfetti, 1985; Samuels, 1987; Stanovich, 1993; Sticht & James, 1984; Wiig, Semel, & Crouse, 1973).

This chapter provides an overview of one major component of a comprehensive intervention approach. Metacognitive strategies designed to increase the scope and utilization of central resources are described in the following sections. This chapter is an abridged chapter (Chermak & Musiek, 1997), with the original chapter including metalinguistic strategies. The reader is reminded, however, that metalinguistic and metacognitive strategies training should be implemented in conjunction with auditory process training and signal quality enhancement, with ample collaboration among professionals (e.g., audiologists, educators, speech-language pathologists) and families to realize a powerful and effective comprehensive management approach.

METACOGNITIVE KNOWLEDGE AND STRATEGIES

Although some central auditory processes may be difficult to change, comprehension of spoken language can be improved by developing better strategies. Effective listeners generally use various strategies to guide information processing and synthesis of the spoken message. Since the metacognitive components trained (i.e., planning, checking, and monitoring) are not task specific, but rather constitute a general strategy for problem solving, the likelihood for generalization of strategy use to other appropriate situations is excellent (Brown, Campione, & Barclay, 1979; Lodico, Ghatala, Levin, Pressley, & Bell, 1983). Interventions combining performance strategies (e.g., using context to derive word meaning, invoking schema to guide interpretation) plus self-control training are likely to be more successful than either approach in isolation (Brown, Campione, & Day, 1981). As illustrated in the following sections, aspects of one metacognitive approach often reinforce elements undergirding a related metacognitive approach. For instance, motivation is fundamental to assertiveness training and attribution training strengthens motivation. Hence, effective treatment programs will likely include a number of metacognitive (i.e., self-control) strategies coupled with appropriate performance strategies.

Several metacognitive approaches may be incorporated in CAPD management programs. Notwithstanding differences among these approaches, they promote active self-regulation and share in common several features. Typically, they provide explicit and detailed instruction regarding the goals of strategies and their application to tasks, as well as training self-regulation and self-monitoring of strategy deployment and outcomes of that deployment (Palincsar & Brown, 1987). They encourage self-identification of strategies employed and the rationale for their use, as well as feedback about the efficacy of strategies for particular tasks (Palincsar & Brown, 1987; Pressley, Borkowski, & O'Sullivan, 1984).

Four metacognitive approaches useful in managing CAPD are discussed next. They are attribution training, cognitive behavior modification, reciprocal teaching, and assertiveness training.

ATTRIBUTION TRAINING

Attribution training targets motivation. Individuals with CAPD are at risk for developing motivational problems as a consequence of chronic listening problems, the often associated academic or workplace failures, and the social frustrations resulting from decreased ability to integrate in a peer group or in one's family. Some individuals become reconciled to the belief that their listening abilities (and perhaps intellectual abilities as well) are poor and cannot be improved, and their efforts to succeed are futile. These beliefs lead to poor motivation and a deterioration in task persistence when faced with challenging listening tasks and conditions (Torgesen, 1980).

Attribution (re)training is undertaken to instill causal attributions for failure to factors that are under the individual's control (e.g., insufficient effort) rather than sensory or intellectual incapacity. It provides a direct approach to reestablish self-confidence and persistence in individuals who present a maladaptive motivational pattern (Licht & Kistner, 1986). Even though children younger than 7 to 10 years are less like to attribute failure to incapacity (Eshel & Klein, 1981; Rholes, Blackwell, Jordan, & Walters, 1980; Stipek, 1981; Stipek & Tannatt, 1984), incorporating attribution training in therapy programs for young children with CAPD offers a preventive approach to motivational problems.

Basically a two-step process, the client is confronted with some failure (e.g., incorrect response to a question posed following an oral-aural story presentation) in the first phase. In the second phase, the clinician induces the client to attribute the failure to insufficient effort. For example, in response to the client who incorrectly responds to a question, the clinician might tell the client that his or her answer was not correct and that although he or she is working hard, even more careful listening is needed. Likewise, successes should be attributed to effort, providing feedback that communicates that the response was correct and acknowledging that the client was listening carefully and trying hard.

The wording of attributional statements is key to the success of this method. Feedback acknowledging hard work and the efforts already expended, while urging even greater effort, should motivate the client and result in improved performance and enhanced self-efficacy (Miller, Brickman, & Bolen, 1975; Schunk, 1982). In addition to the specific wording of the attributional statements, the proportion of successes and failures and the scheduling of failures also influence the effectiveness of attribution retraining. Although confronting failure is integral to attribution retraining, a moderate amount of success is necessary to establish a belief in the method's premise that increased effort will lead to increased success (Clifford, 1978; Dweck, 1975).

Perhaps most important, attribution retraining must be credible. The validity of the new attributions can be established only if the increased effort does, in fact, lead to improved performance (Dweck, 1977). The full complement of metacognitive and metalinguistic strategies must be available to the client and must be coupled with attribution retraining to maximize the chances that additional effort will lead to improved performance (Reid & Borkowski, 1987).

COGNITIVE BEHAVIOR MODIFICATION

Cognitive behavior modification promotes active, self-regulatory listening and learning styles. The goal of cognitive behavior modification is to induce self-control through a planful, reflective processing and response style (Lloyd, 1980). The client is instructed in the use of a strategy, including how to employ, monitor, check, and evaluate that strategy (Brown et al., 1981).

Although classified into four categories (i.e., self-instruction, problem solving, self-regulation, and cognitive strategy training), cognitive behavior modification procedures share a number of features. They each involve clients as active collaborators in the clinical process, include modeling of the target strategy during training, focus on a reflective processing and response style, and emphasize the relationship between the client's actions and task outcomes (Lloyd, 1980; Meichenbaum, 1986). Revealing both the common and divergent foci of the four cognitive behavior modification approaches, self-instruction employs directive self-statements to train task-specific strategies and self-control, whereas cognitive strategy training focuses on the former and self-regulation training emphasizes the latter. Cognitive problem solving procedures incorporate self-instruction, self-monitoring, and self-regulation techniques; however, these procedures are focused on reducing uncertainty and resolving problems.

Procedures from more than one method often are combined to augment training effectiveness (Whitman, Burgio, & Johnson, 1984). For example, Meichenbaum and Goodman's (1971) five-step self-instruction program may be employed across cognitive behavior training regimens. The use of daily logs or diaries is also common to the procedures. Encouraging the client to maintain a daily log that reflects his or her difficult listening situations and the relative value of strategies deployed to enhance listening promotes self-monitoring of the effectiveness of listening comprehension strategies. A brief discussion of four cognitive behavior modification approaches follows.

Self-Instruction

Self-instruction is focused on training clients to formulate adaptive and self-directing verbal statements before and during a task or situation. Five sequential steps comprise self-instruction:

1. Task performance by the clinician while self-verbalizing aloud
2. Performance by the client while the clinician verbalizes
3. Performance by the client while self-instructing aloud
4. Performance by the client while whispering
5. Performance by the client while self-instructing covertly (Meichenbaum & Goodman, 1971)

Training self-instruction by progressing through Meichenbaum and Goodman's five-step approach should promote learning and generalization of the self-instructional routine.

Several problem-solving skills are incorporated in self-instruction, as illustrated in Figure 4.1. Steps 1 and 2 elicit planful, reflective responding. Step 2 also focuses the client's attention on relevant aspects of the task. Steps 3, 4, and 5 involve problem solving. The clinician may encourage general or, as in the case illustrated in Figure 4.1, more specific problem-solving self-instructions, depending on the nature of the

FIGURE 4.1   Self-Instruction: Steps and Statements

Attend, Plan, Reflect

1. How do I listen carefully? I have to pay attention. I must not let myself become distracted. I must listen for important key words as well as content.
2. What is the primary purpose of this message? To tell a story? To describe an event? To explain? To argue a point?

Problem Solving

3. What key words have been stated? What do these key words tell me?
4. What about the context? What experience do I bring to this message?
5. What is the main message? What predictions or inferences are appropriate?

Monitoring, Evaluation, and Feedback

6. Are my conclusions, predictions, and inferences correct? Do they follow from the spoken words? Are they logical?
7. Yes, they are correct. I am an effective listener.

task. Clients should be challenged to ask more sophisticated questions, demanding higher-level thinking commensurate with the message content and task requirements (Wilson, Lanza, & Barton, 1988). Self-monitoring and feedback are provided in step 6. If the client is not successful, it is helpful to include some strategy for coping with failure in step 6. Self-reinforcement, the final step in the self-instruction routine, instills a sense of pride and accomplishment and should increase the client's motivation to transfer the self-instructional technique to novel situations.

Cognitive Problem Solving

Cognitive problem solving offers a systematic process that leads clients to resolve problem situations. It is a five-stage process in which the clinician serves as a consultant as the client learns a self-control technique (Haaga & Davison, 1986).

Clients with CAPD can be taught to treat the spoken message as a problem to be solved by deploying metacognitive processes in conjunction with the requisite auditory and language skills. They are taught to analyze situations and generate a variety of potentially viable responses, recognizing and implementing the most effective response. Further, they are helped to confront cognitive distortions (e.g., catastrophizing, jumping to conclusions) that may be producing unnecessary anxiety or fear (Hart & Morgan, 1993). Self-regulation procedures (described in the next section) are used to maintain and generalize the productive response (Goldfried & Davison, 1976).

The clinician may model problem solving using Meichenbaum and Goodman's (1971) self-instruction program, outlined in the preceding section. Problem solving begins with preparation, or familiarizing oneself with the nature of the problem. The second stage requires the generation of hypotheses regarding solutions to the problem. In the third stage, one evaluates the solution options, considers their utility and predicts possible costs or consequences, and selects the best one. The fourth stage is bifurcated. If a viable solution is found, it is implemented; if no solution is deemed tenable, the incubation phase begins, during which no active effort is expended toward solving the problem (Halpern, 1984). Ironically, it is during this phase that solutions often appear *out of the blue* (Halpern, 1984, p. 163). A fifth stage in the process involves the monitoring and evaluation of one's performance in relation to solving the problem. Self-monitoring homework assignments are useful in measuring progress. Self-reinforcement for successful problem solving (e.g., spoken language understanding) should lead to enhanced self-efficacy and generalization of the process (Haaga & Davison, 1986).

Self-Regulation Procedures

The goal of self-regulation training is self-control (Brown et al., 1981; Whitman et al., 1984). A three-stage training process—involving self-monitoring, self-evaluation, and self-reinforcement—begins by increasing awareness of the behavior targeted for control and proceeds by teaching goal setting and self-monitoring skills for behavioral change (Kanfer & Gaelick, 1986; Whitman et al., 1984). Self-regulation training promotes effective listening by encouraging the listener to monitor comprehension processes to determine whether they are meeting his or her comprehension needs. Upon detecting comprehension errors, disruptions, or inadequacies, the listener learns to modify strategies to handle ambiguities, inconsistencies, or complexities that might otherwise compromise spoken language understanding (Danks & End, 1987).

Cognitive Strategy Training

Cognitive strategy training teaches specific strategies underlying effective performance (Brown & French, 1979). The goal is to help clients become skilled in the use of task strategies and more aware of their own cognitive processes (Whitman et al., 1984). Extended strategy training and feedback on the strategy's effectiveness are crucial to successful implementation of cognitive strategy training (Whitman et al., 1984). Strategies may be trained following Meichenbaum and Goodman's (1971) five-step self-instruction program, outlined previously.

RECIPROCAL TEACHING

Following from the adage that people learn best that which they teach, reciprocal teaching involves alternating roles between the client and clinician, allowing the client to assume the role of teacher as well as student (Casanova, 1989; Chermak, Curtis, & Seikel, 1996; Palincsar & Brown, 1984). In addition to its potential to boost self-esteem and self-efficacy, reciprocal teaching is a highly motivating technique that provides an excellent opportunity for clients to anchor their metacognitive process knowledge by making explicit their knowledge and use of strategies. Reciprocal teaching has been used effectively in a number of areas, including reading comprehension, self-monitoring, memory, and health education, including hearing conservation (Chermak et al., 1996; Clarke, MacPherson, Holmes, & Jones, 1986; Palincsar & Brown, 1984, 1986; Paris, Wixson, & Palincsar, 1986).

Reciprocal teaching is based on the following principles and procedures:

1. The clinician-teacher actively models the desired behavior, making the processing strategies overt, explicit, and concrete.
2. The strategies are modeled in context.
3. Discussions focus on the content of the message as well as the client's understanding of the strategies being used for message comprehension.
4. The clinician provides feedback appropriate to the client's level of mastery.
5. Responsibility for comprehension is transferred from the clinician to the client as soon as the client demonstrates an adequate success level (Harris & Sipay, 1990).

Reciprocal teaching can be expanded to include peer tutoring.

Cognitive Style and Reasoning

Effective listening requires reasoning to critically evaluate and ultimately reconstruct the messages one hears. Flexibility to invoke the cognitive style that best meets changing task demands is necessary to ensure accurate and efficient processing. Inflexible reasoning and sole reliance on any one cognitive style is ineffective in meeting the variety of processing demands and listening tasks, especially given the imprecision and ambiguity inherent to acoustic (e.g., auditory illusions such as phonemic restoration and verbal transformation effects) and linguistic signals (e.g., polysemy, figurative language such as metaphors, idioms, and proverbs). The inadequacy of a single cognitive style can be seen in the failure to infer due to overreliance on literal interpretation. This overreliance leads to misunderstanding a message's content. Similarly, overreliance on a top-down processing style may cause schema inflexibility, biasing interpretation and impeding comprehension.

The importance of accessing multiple cognitive styles is amplified for persons with CAPD whose deficient auditory processes render them less able to cope with degraded acoustic signals and for whom sole reliance on bottom-up processing would leave them extremely vulnerable to comprehension problems. Cognitive style is subject to change through training. For example, children become more reflective following training in the use of a verbal self-control strategy (Craighead, Wilcoxon-Craighead, & Meyers, 1978). Although clients with CAPD are trained to take advantage of information revealed through bottom-up processing (e.g., auditory discrimination, including changes in prosody), one should also emphasize the benefits of top-down processing for *reading between the lines,* recognizing conceptual nuances, reaching auditory and grammatic closure, and inferring or abstracting meaning.

Given the importance of cognitive style flexibility for spoken language comprehension and the opportunity for change, instruction promoting cognitive flexibility should benefit individuals with CAPD. Such instruction may include inferencing skills, which can be developed through the context-derived, vocabulary-building technique described earlier and through the use of short stories that require inferencing on the basis of perceptual information, logic, and/or evidence. Children's poetry requiring inferencing for interpretation can be read to younger children and discussed. In addition to promoting cognitive-style flexibility, inferencing also challenges memory, as stored knowledge is essential to the inferencing process. Attention to the appropriate use of other cognitive styles (e.g., divergent/convergent, impulsive/reflective, adaptive/innovative, synthetic/analytic, field dependent/field independent) should also be introduced in therapy.

ASSERTIVENESS TRAINING

Assertion is "self-expression through which one stands up for one's own basic human rights without violating the basic human rights of others" (Kelley, 1979, p. 14). The goal of assertion is to attain personal effectiveness by communicating that which one feels, thinks, and wants. Assertive behavior is self-enhancing and empowering, and it furthers attainment of desired goals (Alberti & Emmons, 1978). Although assertiveness can be learned (Bornstein, Bellack, & Hersen, 1977; Rehm,

Fuchs, Roth, Kornblith, & Romano, 1979), self-confidence and self-esteem are prerequisite (Kelley, 1979). Moreover, motivation drives asser-tiveness: Without a desire to succeed, one is unlikely to assume personal responsibility inherent to assertiveness. Similarly, command of basic interpersonal and communication skills is necessary to effective asser-tiveness. Since assertive clients tend to be more actively involved in plan-ning and directing their own therapy, they tend to derive greater gain. Moreover, they tend to generalize new strategies and skills to everyday life contexts.

Integral to assertion are verbal and nonverbal skills and a positive cognitive *mindset* (Kelley, 1979). Assertion typically involves a verbal exchange; the individual must formulate and deliver an assertive mes-sage (Kelley, 1979). In addition to the actual words used to express the assertion, the effectiveness of the assertion will be influenced by the non-verbal aspects of the message's delivery. A positive cognitive set rein-forces one's confidence in the value and right to assert and motivates one to persist (Kelley, 1979). Assertiveness training techniques may involve modeling, guided practice, coaching, homework and self-management, readings, and small group discussions (Kelley, 1979). Related anxiety-reduction techniques include relaxation, imagery, self-talk, coping, and desensitization (Kendall, 1992).

SUMMARY

A comprehensive management approach is necessary to improve listen-ing ability and spoken language comprehension by individuals with central auditory processing disorders. This chapter focused on one major component of such a comprehensive approach—self-regulation of lin-guistic, cognitive, and metacognitive strategies. These strategies assist the listener in structuring auditory input, guiding information process-ing, and understanding spoken language. Facility with these strategies should allow for generalization of effective listening skills across settings.

REFERENCES

Alberti, R. E., & Emmons, M. L. (1978). *Your perfect right* (3rd ed.). San Luis Obispo, CA: Impact.

American Speech-Language-Hearing Association: Task Force on Central Audi-tory Processing Concensus Development. (1996). Central auditory process-ing: Current status of research and implications for clinical practice. *American Journal of Audiology, 5*(2), 41–54.

Bornstein, M. R., Bellack, A. S., & Hersen, M. (1977). Social-skills training for unassertive children: A multiple-baseline analysis. *Journal of Applied Behavior Analysis, 10,* 183–195.

Brown, A. L., Campione, J., & Barclay, C. R. (1979). Training self-checking routines for estimating test readiness: Generalization for list learning to prose recall. *Child Development, 50,* 501–512.

Brown, A. L., Campione, J. C., & Day, J. D. (1981). Learning to learn: On training students to learn from texts. *Educational Researcher, 10,* 14–21.

Brown, A. L., & French, L. (1979). The zone of potential development: Implications for intelligence testing in the year 2000. *Intelligence, 2,* 46–53.

Casanova, U. (1989). Being the teacher helps students learn. *Instructor, 98*(9), 12–13.

Chermak, G. D., Curtis, L., & Seikel, J. A. (1996). The effectiveness of an interactive hearing conservation program for elementary school children. *Language, Speech, and Hearing Services in Schools, 27*(1), 29–39.

Chermak, G. D., & Musiek, F. E. (1992). Managing central auditory processing disorders in children and youth. *American Journal of Audiology, 1*(3), 61–65.

Chermak, G. D., & Musiek, F. E. (1997). *Central auditory processing disorders: New perspectives.* San Diego: Singular.

Clarke, J., MacPherson, B., Holmes, D., & Jones, R. (1986). Reducing adolescent smoking: A comparison of peer-led, teacher-led, and expert interventions. *Journal of School Health, 98*(2), 92–96.

Clifford, M. M. (1978). Have we underestimated the facilitative effects of failure? *Canadian Journal of Behavioral Science, 10,* 308–316.

Craighead, W. E., Wilcoxon-Craighead, L., & Meyers, A. (1978). New directions in behavior modification with children. In M. Hersen, R. Eisler, & P. Miller (Eds.), *Progress in behavior modification* (Vol. 6, pp. 159–201). New York: Academic Press.

Danks, J. H., & End, L. J. (1987). Processing strategies for reading and listening. In R. Horowitz & S. J. Samuels (Eds.), *Comprehending oral and written language* (pp. 271–294). San Diego, CA: Academic Press.

Dweck, C. S. (1975). The role of expectations and attributions in the alleviation of learned helplessness. *Journal of Personality and Social Psychology, 31,* 674–685.

Dweck, C. S. (1977). Learned helplessness and negative evaluation. *The Educator, 14,* 44–49.

Eshel, Y., & Klein, Z. (1981). Development of academic self-concept of lower-class and middle-class primary school children. *Journal of Educational Psychology, 73,* 287–293.

Goldfried, M. R., & Davison, G. C. (1976). *Clinical behavior therapy.* New York: Holt, Rinehart and Winston.

Haaga, D. A., & Davison, G. C. (1986). Cognitive change methods. In F. H. Kanfer & A. P. Goldstein (Eds.), *Helping people change: A textbook of methods* (pp. 236–282). New York: Pergamon Press.

Halpern, D. F. (1984). *Thought and knowledge: An introduction to critical thinking.* Hillsdale, NJ: Lawrence Erlbaum.

Harris, A. J., & Sipay, E. R. (1990). *How to increase reading ability* (9th ed.). New York: Longman. London: Academic Press.

Hart, K. J., & Morgan, J. R. (1993). Cognitive-behavioral procedures with children: Historical context and current status. In A. J. Finch, W. M. Nelson, & E. S. Ott (Eds.), *Cognitive-behavioral procedures with children and adolescents* (p. 124). Boston: Allyn and Bacon.

Kanfer, F. H., & Gaelick, L. (1986). Self-management methods. In F. H. Kanfer & A. P. Goldstein (Eds.), *Helping people change: A textbook of methods* (3rd ed., pp. 283–345). New York: Pergamon Press.

Kelley, C. (1979). *Assertion training: A facilitator's guide.* San Diego: University Associates.

Kendall, P. C. (1992). *Anxiety disorders in youth.* Boston: Allyn and Bacon.

Licht, B., & Kistner, J. A. (1986). Motivational problems of learning-disabled children: Individual differences and their implications for treatment. In J. K. Torgesen & B. Y. L. Wong (Eds.), *Psychological and educational perspectives on learning disabilities* (pp. 225–255). San Diego: Academic Press.

Lloyd, J. (1980). Academic instruction and cognitive behavior modification: The need for attack strategy training. *Exceptional Education Quarterly, 1*, 53–64.

Lodico, M. G., Ghatala, E. S., Levin, J. R., Pressley, M., & Bell, J. A. (1983). The effects of strategy monitoring training on children's selection of effective memory strategies. *Journal of Experimental Child Psychology, 35*, 263–277.

Meichenbaum, D. (1986). Cognitive-behavior management. In F. H. Kanfer & A. P. Goldstein (Eds.), *Helping people change: A textbook of methods* (3rd ed., pp. 346–380). New York: Pergamon Press.

Meichenbaum, D., & Goodman, J. (1971). Training impulsive children to talk to themselves: A means of developing self-control. *Journal of Abnormal Psychology, 77*, 115–126.

Miller, R. L., Brickman, P., & Bolen, D. (1975). Attribution versus persuasion as a means for modifying behavior. *Journal of Personality and Social Psychology, 31*, 430–441.

Palincsar, A. S., & Brown, A. L. (1984). Reciprocal teaching of comprehension fostering and comprehension monitoring activities. *Cognition and Instruction, 1*, 117–175.

Palincsar, A. S., & Brown, A. L. (1986). Interactive teaching to promote independent learning from text. *Reading Teacher, 39*, 771–771.

Palincsar, A. S., & Brown, A. L. (1987). Enhancing instructional time through attention to metacognition. *Journal of Learning Disabilities, 20*, 66–75.

Paris, S. G., Wixson, K. K., & Palincsar, A. S. (1986). Instructional approaches to reading comprehension. In E. Z. Rothkopf (Ed.), *Review of research on education* (Vol. 13, pp. 91–218). Washington, DC: American Educational Research Association.

Perfetti, C.A. (1985). *Reading ability.* New York: Oxford University Press.

Pressley, M., Borkowski, J. G., & O'Sullivan, J. T. (1984). Memory strategy instruction is made of this: Metamemory and durable strategy use. *Educational Psychologist, 19*, 94–107.

Rehm, L. P., Fuchs, C. Z., Roth, D. M., Kornblith, S. I., & Romano, J. M. (1979). A comparison of self-control and assertion skills treatments of depression. *Behavior Therapy, 10,* 429–442.

Reid, M. K., & Borkowski, J. G. (1987). Causal attributions of hyperactive children: Implications for training strategies and self-control. *Journal of Educational Psychology, 76,* 225–235.

Rholes, W. S., Blackwell, J., Jordan, C., & Walters, C. (1980). A developmental study of learned helplessness. *Developmental Psychology, 16,* 616–624.

Samuels, S. J. (1987). Factors that influence listening and reading comprehension. In R. Horowitz & S. J. Samuels (Eds.), *Comprehending oral and written language* (pp. 295–325). San Diego: Academic Press.

Schunk, D. H. (1982). Effects of effort attributional feedback on children's perceived self-efficacy and achievement. *Journal of Educational Psychology, 74,* 548–556.

Stanovich, K. E. (1993). The construct validity of discrepancy definitions of reading disability. In G. R. Lyon, D. B. Gray, J. F. Kavanaugh, & N. A. Krasnegor (Eds.), *Better understanding learning disabilities* (pp. 273–307). Baltimore: Paul H. Brookes.

Sticht, T. G., & James, J. H. (1984). Listening and reading. In P. D. Pearson (Ed.), *Handbook of reading research* (pp. 293–317). New York: Longman.

Stipek, D. J. (1981). Children's perceptions of their own and their classmates' ability. *Journal of Educational Psychology, 73,* 404–410.

Stipek, D. J., & Tannatt, L. M. (1984). Children's judgments of their own and their peers' academic competence. *Journal of Educational Psychology, 76,* 75–84.

Torgesen, J. K. (1980). Conceptual and educational implications of the use of efficient task strategies by learning disabled children. *Journal of Learning Disabilities, 13,* 364–371.

Whitman, T. L., Burgio, L., & Johnson, M. B. (1984). Cognitive behavioral interventions with mentally retarded children. In A. Meyers & W. E. Craighead (Eds.), *Cognitive behavior therapy with children* (pp. 193–227). New York: Plenum Press.

Wiig, E. H., Semel, E. M., & Crouse, M. A. B. (1973). The use of morphology by high risk and learning disabled children. *Journal of Learning Disabilities, 7,* 457–465.

Wilson, C. C., Lanza, J. R., & Barton, J. S. (1988). Developing higher level thinking skills through questioning techniques in the speech and language setting. *Language, Speech and Hearing Services in Schools, 19,* 428–431.

5

MEMORY AND ATTENTION PROCESSING DEFICITS

A Guide to Management Strategies

LARRY MEDWETSKY
Rochester Hearing and Speech Center

The primary focus of this chapter is to inform the reader of management strategies for addressing memory and attention deficits in spoken language perception. Selecting the appropriate management strategies is not straightforward and may involve assessing processes not typically considered. To successfully address these deficits, clinicians must be aware of (1) the underlying memory and attention processes employed in spoken language perception, (2) the types of breakdowns that can occur, and, in turn, (3) choose the appropriate strategies to address these deficits. A number of topics will be addressed in this chapter, including:

1. Capacity and load
2. Memory and attentional processes of spoken language perception
3. Memory/attentional deficits and associated management strategies

After reading this chapter, the reader will have a better understanding of the complexity of spoken language perception and will feel more confident in managing memory and attention deficits.

CAPACITY AND LOAD

An individual's ability to complete a task successfully can be reduced to the relationship between two variables: capacity and load. *Capacity* is defined as the total reservoir of energy that an individual has available to expend on a particular task, and *load* refers to the amount of energy actually expended on that task. Figure 5.1 summarizes this relationship; the outer circle represents capacity, and the inner circle represents load. The arrows indicate that both capacity and load can increase or decrease. An individual will successfully complete a task as long as the load is less than the individual's capacity for that particular task; however, if the load exceeds the individual's capacity, then difficulty and possible failure on that task would likely ensue.

An individual's capacity for a particular task is determined by a number of variables, including (1) inherent physical attributes, (2) environmental influences, and (3) degree of arousal. The following example elaborates on these concepts:

> Joe Smith is set to attempt a new world's record in the bench press. He has been weightlifting over 10 years and has developed his physique and technique to the point where he appears ready to complete this task successfully. He is "psyching" himself for the task. He lifts the weight and is _____.

FIGURE 5.1   The Interrelationship between Capacity and Load

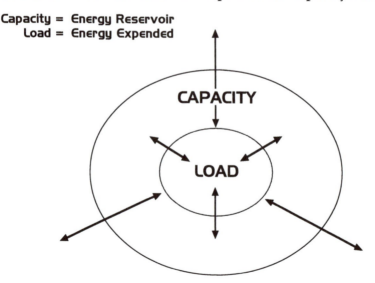

In this example, Joe Smith brings forth to this task certain inherent physical attributes. For weightlifting, his inherited body attributes (including the number of muscle cells and muscle cell size) play an important role in determining the total amount he may ever lift. However, environmental influences can also significantly influence an individual's success on a task. In weightlifting, this would consist of a rigorous training regimen for increasing muscle mass and proper weightlifting techniques. Last, an individual's arousal level has a significant impact on performance; in weightlifting, a person would be expected to perform at his optimum if he was refreshed and not stressed.

Figure 5.2 illustrates the relationship between performance level and arousal level. Individuals achieve maximum performance at moderate arousal level—that is, when they are fresh and relaxed. However, when individuals are fatigued or bored, their arousal levels decrease; this, in turn, would result in a concomitant drop in performance. On the other hand, if individuals were to become significantly stressed or frozen with fear, as may happen in the face on an oncoming car, arousal levels would increase significantly and result in decreased performance (in this scenario, possible immobility and being struck by the car).

FIGURE 5.2   The Relationship between Performance Level and Arousal Level

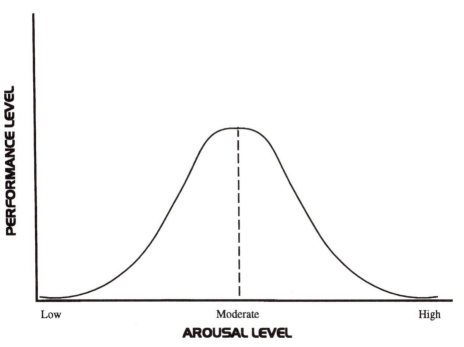

The load required by a particular task can also change over time. The example provided here will be familiar to most readers:

> When Susan Miller was learning to drive, she had a great deal to remember. She had to learn how to steer, brake, look in the different mirrors, and remember which traffic signs stood for what. And pity the person who dared to talk to her while she was driving.
> [One year later] Susan has just arrived at work and is getting out of her mini-van. "Strange," Susan thought, "I can't recall the roads that I have just driven on to get to work."

This example illustrates how, through repetition, a task can become so automatic that the mental load entailed by that task decreases dramatically. Note that this does not mean that the load entailed by driving has been permanently reduced. For example:

> One day when it was raining hard and Susan's four kids were screaming in the back of the van, she had such a hard time driving she almost hit another car.

In this case, the load increased so much that it almost exceeded the individual's capacity and she almost had an accident.

When load is discussed in spoken language perception, one typically refers to an individual's mental workload—that is, the amount of mental energy expended on a task (Kahneman, 1973; Gopher & Donchin; 1986). Numerous factors determine the mental workload expended, including (1) the listener's familiarity with the task and stimuli, (2) the amount of information that must be processed over a specific time period, (3) the discriminability of the stimulus, and (4) the amount of "noise" embedded in the stimulus (these will be elaborated on in subsequent sections). Hence, the extent to which mental energy must be expended, as well as the perceiver's capacity to process the information, determines whether the listener will process spoken language stimuli successfully.

MEMORY AND ATTENTIONAL PROCESSES OF SPOKEN LANGUAGE PERCEPTION

This discussion describes the various memory and attentional processes employed in auditory spoken language perception. The information presented is based on an information-processing model approach (Massaro, 1975; Massaro & Cohen, 1975; Klatzky, 1984; Gregg, 1986; Hawkins &

Presson, 1986; Wyer & Srull, 1989). An *information-processing model* attempts to conceptualize the various memory structures and psychological processes presumed to operate between the onset of the stimulus and an individual's response. Massaro (1975) defines *memory structures* as storage components that hold information. *Psychological processes* are operations that involve the transformation from one memory structure to another. Because the listener is limited in the amount of information he or she can retain in short-term "conscious" memory, two important processes are engaged. One process is that of attention—the ability to focus selectively on the stimuli of interest and ignore irrelevant competing stimuli, thereby limiting the amount of information processed to resolution. The second process involves the ability to recode information into even larger chunks; that is, at successively higher stages in processing, increasingly greater amounts of information are contained per unit (Miller, 1956). For example, the letters *C-A-T* or *D-O-G* consist of three chunks of information. However, over time, an individual learns to recode the letters into one unit, thus increasing the amount of information contained per unit.

Figure 5.3 highlights the author's conceptualization of the main components of the auditory information-processing model. The boxes represent memory structures and the arrows represent psychological processes. In the first stage, the acoustic stimulus is first transformed mechanically, hydraulically, and electrically via the middle ear, cochlea, and central auditory nervous system. Features such as intensity, frequency, and timing are extracted from the electrical representations. However, because recognition of an auditory stimulus is not immediate, it must somehow be stored; this is thought to occur in *preperceptual acous-*

FIGURE 5.3   The Author's Conceptualization of the Main Components of Auditory Information Processing

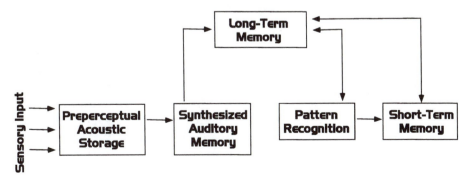

tic storage, often referred to as *echoic memory* (Massaro, 1975; Massaro & Cohen, 1975; Gregg, 1986; Hawkins & Presson, 1986). The importance of the echoic memory stage is that it enables the listener to continue processing a signal no longer in physical existence. Results from various studies show that an individual's ability to extract featural information increases steadily up to 250 milliseconds after onset (Massaro, 1970, 1972; Massaro & Cohen, 1975; Hawkins & Presson, 1986; Gregg, 1986).

In the next stage, the featural content in preperceptual auditory storage is combined and transformed into a percept that is stored in *synthesized auditory memory* (Massaro, 1975). This stage allows an individual to characterize incoming stimuli on the basis of such characteristics as spatial location, intonation, and intensity. That is, even if further processing of the signal was to be disrupted, an individual would still be able to identify the location, pitch, or loudness of a signal but not the linguistic content.

It should be noted that Massaro (1976) found that attentional mechanisms do not affect performance in the echoic memory stage. However, attention does greatly influence performance for synthesized auditory memory and subsequent stages of processing. That is, for intervals greater than 250 milliseconds after signal offset, attention can significantly enhance the processing of target stimuli.

The next stage involves the psychological process known as *pattern recognition.* Massaro (1975, 1976) proposed that the synthesized auditory percepts (i.e., the combination of physical features) are then compared to stored patterns in long-term memory. Perceptual identification and interpretation result from the best match. The activation of the stored percepts from long-term memory appears to depend on the interaction of a number of factors, including the following:

1. Activation threshold of the unit stored in long-term memory
2. Subject's expectations
3. Linguistic and "world" context
4. Amount of focal attention given to that particular stimulus
5. Strength and discriminability of the stimulus

It is believed that units stored in long-term memory have different activation thresholds (Norman, 1979; Kahneman, 1973; Klatzky, 1984). For example, some stored units have lower thresholds and are more readily activated than others. Note that these activation thresholds are quasi-permanent in nature but can be altered over time by *repeated exposure,* since well-learned patterns have lower activation thresholds than those involving infrequent stimulation. Thresholds may also be lowered because of emotional importance (e.g., one's name).

In addition, activation thresholds can also be altered on a momentary basis as a result of (1) listener's expectations (stored units corresponding with a listener's expectations will exhibit momentarily decreased thresholds), (2) linguistic context (syntax, semantic content) and social context (topic, body language), and (3) focal attention given to that particular stimulus (attention will excite and lower the activation thresholds of those stored units corresponding to the target stimuli).

Another variable determining whether a stored percept will be activated from long-term memory involves stimulus intensity; that is, stimuli significantly above a subject's threshold are more likely to activate the corresponding prototype from long-term memory. A related variable is that of the discriminability of a speech stimulus. *Discriminability* refers to the presence or absence of salient feature components within a stimulus. That is, it is easier for individuals to identify the stimulus if the processed featural components of that stimulus are fairly complete. For example, individuals with a high frequency hearing loss will exhibit difficulty in extracting many important acoustic cues from the signal, which, in turn, will make it harder for individuals to match the stimuli accurately with the corresponding stored units in long-term memory.

The last stage, prior to a subject initiating a response, is *short-term memory*, also known as *working memory*. Short-term memory is thought to be the stage where the information just processed or that retrieved from long-term memory is within an individual's conscious awareness. Short-term memory is limited both in capacity and time, whereas long-term memory is essentially unlimited. One measure of short-term memory is an individual's *span of apprehension*, also known as *short-term memory span*. Short-term memory span refers to the maximum number of units processed and retained at any one point in time. Factors affecting short-term memory span include the following:

1. Familiarity of stimuli
2. Utilization of rehearsal strategies
3. Articulatory difficulty of stimuli
4. Schema organization in long-term memory
5. Suprasegmental information (e.g., intonation, stress patterns, and pauses)
6. Attentional allocation

Familiarity of Stimuli

Miller (1956) found that adult short-term memory span for familiar material such as digits and household objects is on the order of 7 ± 2 units. He also found that short-term memory span dropped significantly when listeners were presented with less familiar items. This drop in performance may be related to the increased energy and time of processing that must be expended in matching unfamiliar stimuli with stored prototypes before the latter can be activated from long-term memory.

Rehearsal Strategies

The importance of rehearsal strategies is that they maintain and slow down the decay of items stored in working memory. Rehearsal reinforces the continued presence of target stimuli in short-term memory. In spoken language perception, items are subject to rapid loss from short-term store; however, this loss can be delayed by means of rehearsal. An example of rehearsal is when an individual needs to make a phone call and is told a telephone number. If the individual repeats the numbers to himself, he will usually be successful in retaining them in memory until he can dial the number. However, if the individual is unable to rehearse these numbers, such as if he is distracted, then he will be unable to recall more than just a few of these numbers.

Articulatory Difficulty

Another factor affecting short-term memory span is the articulatory difficulty of items (Baddeley, Thomson, & Buchanan, 1975). Baddeley and colleagues found that the number of words recalled varied as a function of articulatory difficulty (note that word *frequency* was taken into account in this study). Since rehearsal usually involves repeating items silently to oneself, it would be expected that difficult-to-pronounce items would adversely affect rehearsal, and, in turn, result in a decreased short-term memory span for these items. However, this author has not read of any published study that has examined the span of apprehension for individuals with articulatory difficulty, hence, it is unclear as to the generalizability of the results seen by Baddeley and colleagues.

Organization of Schema

A number of researchers have proposed that one component of long-term memory is what has come to be known as *schema* (Rumelhart & Ortony, 1977; Thorndyke, 1977; Norman, 1979). Schema are thought to consist of percepts that preserve relations among its constituent components. For example, a schema of a "zoo" might consist of percepts of the various animals and the scenery typically found in a zoo. It is likely that when stored percepts are activated by incoming stimuli, these activated units, in turn, lower the activation thresholds for other units by which they have become intrinsically linked. Consequently, if schema are well organized, then incoming stimuli will be processed both accurately and efficiently, and quickly transferred to working memory (Norman, 1979).

Suprasegmental Information

The presence of suprasegmental information has been shown to improve listener accuracy, especially in difficult listening conditions (Wingfield, 1975; Collier & Hart, 1975; Brokx & Nooteboom, 1982). Findings from these studies indicate that suprasegmental cues assist the listener in parsing spoken language into its component phrase structures. This helps the listener process more information per chunk, and, in turn, process longer sentences.

Attentional Allocation

Because the human receiver has a limited capacity for processing incoming stimuli (Miller, 1956; Broadbent, 1958; Kahneman; 1973), it has been proposed that the importance of attentional allocation is to limit the amount of information processed at any one time. That is, it allows an individual to focus selectively on a limited amount of information, hence maximizing the extent to which the target information will be processed and stored. Only the information deemed relevant will be attended to and processed.

Terms such as attention deficit disorder (ADD) imply that attention is a unitary process; in fact, however, attention can be allocated in many ways depending on the task. These include:

1. *Preparatory attention:* the decision process whereby the listener chooses which stimuli to attend
2. *Rehearsal:* the ability to maintain and slow down the decay of items stored in working memory
3. *Focused attention:* the ability to attend to a target in quiet or in noise
4. *Sustained attention:* the ability to maintain attention to a target over a period of time
5. *Vigilance:* the ability to maintain preparedness for responding to an intermittent signal (such as the mother of a newborn who can ignore all stimuli while sleeping but will jump to her feet when hearing her baby cry)
6. *Selective attention:* the ability to attend to a target in the face of one or more competing stimuli
7. *Divided attention:* the ability to share attention among two or more target stimuli

Therefore, rather than classifying individuals as being ADD "inattentive type" due to inabilities to focus, stay on task, and so forth, it may be more useful to identify the specific nature of these deficits, which, in turn, would point to the most appropriate management strategies. As mentioned at the onset of this chapter, this can be achieved only if clinicians are aware of the different variables that can have an impact on attention and how to best assess these variables.

It should also be noted that attention is distinct from the memory processes described earlier, in that attention entails conscious decision making processes; that is, the listener consciously selects which stimuli to attend and process. Hence, in evaluating deficits in attention, one should examine both the listener's strategies on a particular listening task (metacognitive skills) as well as perceptual skills.

MEMORY/ATTENTIONAL DEFICITS AND ASSOCIATED MANAGEMENT STRATEGIES

This section will examine (1) factors that can negatively affect the processing of spoken stimuli, (2) the deficits that can ensue, and (3) recommended strategies to address these deficits. (An overview is shown in Table 5.1.)

Initial Processing Stage

Recall that initially stimuli must be stored in echoic memory before any further processing can occur. It is in this stage that acoustic features extracted from the signal are combined into an auditory percept; this ability can be negatively affected by a number of different factors.

Factors Affecting This Stage and Negative Consequences

One important variable is the audibility of acoustic features. Individuals who are hearing impaired obviously have difficulty extracting all of the acoustic features, the extent of this difficulty varying as a function of the degree of hearing loss. However, even people with normal hearing may encounter situations where not all of the acoustic features are audible, such as when they are in noisy surroundings.

In addition to audibility, other factors can negatively affect on accurate feature extraction. These include temporal and frequency resolution. Note that temporal and frequency resolution are not typically measured in the clinic. However, the results from research laboratories have relevance for clinic populations.

TABLE 5.1 Factors Affecting Processing and Management Strategies

Processing Stage	Factors Affecting Stage
1. Echoic Memory/ Feature Extraction	i. Audibility of acoustic features ii. Temporal resolution iii. Frequency resolution iv. Intensity/Phase of signals reaching the ears
2. Pattern Recognition	i. Same as # 1 i, ii, iii. ii. LTM- phoneme/lexicon/schema iii. Semantic relations, syntax iv. Knowledge of world context
3. Short-Term Memory	i. Familiarity of input ii. Organization of prototypes/ schema iii. Articulatory difficulty of items iv. Rehearsal (form of attention) v. Sequencing

4. Attention
  I. Selective Attention (SA)
  II. Divided Attention (DivA)
	i. All factors in # 1, 2, 3
	ii. Attentional allocation (metacognitive skills)
	i. Same as attention but to two or more targets (greater load)
	ii. If must recall more than one target, output interference

(Continued)

TABLE 5.1   (Continued)

Negative Consequences If Deficit Present	Management Strategies
# i, ii, iii. Affects the accurate derivation/internal representation of spoken stimuli iv. Affects binaural integration (such as localization) and separation (important for separating target from competing stimuli)	a. Use (FM) amplification/communication strategies to improve signal-to-noise ratio and audibility for # i–iv b. Phonic approaches (auditory training) and Tallal et al. training approach for ii
ia. Possible difficulty in deriving phonic code, and, in turn, sound-symbol associations ib. Possibly affects receptive language ii. Affects speed/accuracy of decoding and retrieval iii. Affects ability to use language for facilitating predictions (i.e., top-down processing) iv. Affects ability to use world knowledge for facilitating top-down processing	a. Strategies as in # 1a and 1b b. If receptive language is negatively impacted, then one can work on vocabulary building/semantic mapping/syntactic rules and concepts c. Work on pragmatics/world knowledge
i. Longer time to process and retrieve items from LTM ii. Same as # i iii. Same as #i iv. Decreases total time items can be held in STM v. Decreases ability to maintain correct sequence of items/directions	a. Vocabulary building/semantic mapping b. Same as # a c. Speech therapy d. Rehearsal strategies/mnemonics e. Present items/directions one at a time and have client repeat and summarize at end; write down items/directions
i. Breakdown in selective attention ii. Breakdown in divided attention (greater likelihood than selective attention because of greater load)	a. Assistive listening devices/communication strategies, and strategies specific to deficit (as listed above) b. For DivA, same as for SA, but in class, note taker may be useful (for a and b, metacognitive training, if needed)

Temporal resolution refers to the minimum time interval required to segregate or resolve acoustic events. Temporal resolution has been most popularly measured by means of a gap-detection task in which listeners have to detect the presence of a temporal gap in a burst of noise; that is, the smaller the gap that can be detected, the better the temporal resolution. In the hearing impaired, the greater the degree of hearing loss, the poorer the temporal resolution (Pickett, Revoile, & Danaher, 1983; Dorman, 1986). In addition, a number of researchers have shown that individuals with learning/language disorders tend to exhibit poor temporal resolution (Stark & Tallal, 1979; Tallal et al., 1996). A consequence of this poorer temporal resolution is a greater difficulty in resolving various acoustic features for rapidly changing sounds such as place of articulation for stop consonants and third formant information distinguishing the consonant /r/ from /l/.

Frequency resolution refers to an individual's ability to discriminate successive sounds on the basis of frequency. The threshold limen for frequency (i.e., the frequency difference that must exist before an individual can distinguish that the sounds are, in fact, different) is typically larger for listeners who are hearing impaired than in listeners who have normal hearing. As a result, those with hearing impairments, especially those with severe to profound sensorineural hearing loss, tend to exhibit difficulty distinguishing consonants on the basis of frequency information, as well as in resolving formant frequencies in vowels (Pickett, Revoile, & Danaher, 1983; Dorman, 1986; Tyler, 1988).

There are a number of other important consequences resulting from incomplete feature extraction. First, impoverished stimuli are more subject to the effects of backward masking. Subjects presented with a target stimulus followed shortly after by a masking stimulus are less able to recall the target stimulus when acoustic cues have been removed (Pickett, Revoile, & Danaher, 1983). This suggests that individuals who are unable to accurately derive acoustic cues from spoken stimuli are at greater risk for experiencing difficulty in background noise. A second negative consequence of incomplete feature extraction is increased difficulty in deriving accurate phonemic representations.

In addition to feature extraction, sounds can also be characterized on the basis of intensity and phase information reaching the two ears— that is, interaural differences. For example, the localization of sound in space is a binaural phenomenon whereby interaural differences in intensity and phase enable an individual to determine the origin of a particular sound. Because this process requires an internal fusion of the signals reaching both ears, localization is an example of binaural integration. Sounds can also be separated perceptually on the basis of intensity or phase relationships. A classic example of binaural separation is the *masking level difference (MLD)* (Hirsh, 1950; Licklider, 1948). Licklider found that when subjects listened binaurally to both speech and noise of equal intensity under headphones, phase relations between the speech signals and noise masker significantly affected speech intelligibility. In the reference condition, both the speech signal and noise were presented diotically; that is, both signals were presented in phase to the two earphones.

In one test condition, the speech stimuli were presented 180° out of phase to the earphones while the noise was still presented in phase. The magnitude of the improvement in the test condition, was on the order of 10 to 15 dB; that is, in the test condition, subjects were able to achieve similar word recognition scores at a 10 to 15 dB poorer signal-to-noise (S/N) ratio than when both stimuli were presented completely in phase. This improvement in performance is thought to occur in the test condition because the listener perceives the competing stimuli as coming from different regions in perceptual space versus from the same perceptual space in the reference condition. Note that individuals exhibiting reduced MLDs tend to experience increased difficulty in noisy situations. This author assumes that this increased difficulty is due to a reduced ability in separating the target signal from the competing background.

Recommended Management Strategies

If stimuli are inaudible because of a hearing loss, providing amplification is obviously one management option. Hearing aid technology, especially digital aid technology, has advanced to the point where it can enhance spectral features. The use of such technology may one day be extended for individuals who are listening disabled, of course, with little or no amplification. However, hearing aid technology is still unable to address the issues of frequency and temporal resolution.

In addition to hearing aid technology, there are some simple strategies that can be implemented for addressing feature extraction. These include speech reading and preferential seating. *Speech reading* allows many individuals to perceive sounds they might otherwise miss. For example, in noisy bars, even people with normal hearing have difficulty hearing the sounds of speech. One of the ways individuals are able to maintain successful conversation in these difficult listening situations is through speech reading. Although many speech sounds are rendered inaudible in noisy environments, many are quite distinguishable when speech-read. For example, even though weak high-frequency consonants such as /s/, /th/, /f/ may be inaudible to those listening in a noisy environment, individuals usually have little difficulty in distinguishing these sounds through speech reading.

Because the intensity of sound decreases as a function of distance, many speech sounds may become inaudible by the time they reach the listener. Extrapolation of data from various researchers (Ross, 1986; Hawkins, 1984; Boothroyd & Medwetsky, 1992; Boothroyd, Erickson, & Medwetsky, 1994) reveals that the overall sound pressure level (SPL) of speech two inches from the lips is approximately 90 dB, whereas at six feet the overall SPL of speech drops to approximately 65 dB. Therefore, in unfavorable listening environments where both noise and reverberation may have a negative impact on listening, *preferential seating* is often suggested as a strategy for increasing the level of speech sounds reaching the listener. However, there are many situations where preferential seating is not possible. In these instances, the most successful approach to date has involved the use of assistive listening devices (ALDs). Examples of ALDs include FM, infra-red, and induction loop systems. All of these systems consist of a microphone, transmitter, amplifier, and receiver. These systems improve the signal-to-noise ratio essentially by decreasing the distance between the talker and listener. By negating the effects of distance, the intensity of the sound source is maintained at a higher listening level, thereby producing an improved signal-to-noise ratio. The importance of a high signal-to-noise ratio is evident from the research. Individuals who are hearing impaired as well as individuals who are learning disabled perform significantly better when the signal-to-noise ratio is high (Carhart & Tillman, 1970; Finitzo-Hieber & Tillman, 1978; Elliot, 1982; Flexer, Millin, & Brown, 1990).

The following information applies only to those with normal hearing sensitivity. Poor temporal and frequency resolution can have an impact on the accurate derivation and internalization of phonemes (poor phonemic decoding). Thus, management techniques addressing phonemic decoding and synthesis may significantly improve performance. An example of a successful phonics approach is the Auditory Discrimination in Depth program (Lindamood & Lindamood, 1975). This program is used to train individuals to perceive the contrasts between various speech sounds, conceptualize the order of sounds in syllables, and recognize the correspondence between the sequences of sounds in spoken words and sequences of letters in written words. Another training program that is widely used is Phonemic Synthesis: Blending Sounds into Words (Katz & Harmon, 1982). This program has been designed to identify phonemic synthesis difficulties and to provide a practical tool to address phonemic discrimination, sequencing, and blending.

A new tool that shows great promise is a computer interactive program developed by the Keck Center for Integrative Neurosciences and Coleman Laboratory and by the Center for Molecular and Behavioral

Neurosciences, Rutgers University. Recently commercially available through Scientific Learning Corporation, the results in the laboratory have been very encouraging. The development of this computer program is based on much research. Stark and Tallal (1979) found that many children who are language-learning impaired (LLI) exhibit a temporal processing deficit characterized by limited abilities at identifying brief phonemic elements in specific speech contexts and by poor performance in identifying or sequencing short-duration acoustic stimuli presented in rapid succession. When these stimuli have been modified to be presented at slower rates or longer formant transitions, performance improved significantly (Tallal et al., 1996).

The computer program consists of two interactive audiovisual games. The first type uses nonverbal stimuli consisting of frequency-modulated tonal pairs, whereby the sweep frequencies encompass the typical formant transitions of English consonants typically difficult for LLI children (such as stop consonants, third formant transitions in /r/ versus /l/, etc.). The second game involves phonetic element recognition within contrasting consonant-vowel pairs. In both games, stimuli contrasts are altered adaptively, proceeding from the most easily perceived to the direction of normal performance levels. For example, stimuli pairs presented initially may have (1) long interstimulus time intervals, (2) a slow rate of formant transition, or (3) long stimuli durations. Response task also varies in difficulty, ranging from a simple discrimination task (i.e., identifying whether stimuli are the same or different) to identifying speech stimuli in game #2. When a child experiences success at a particular level, the software automatically increases item difficulty. Results have shown that subjects who have undergone this training improve significantly in their ability to identify phonemes.

Pattern Recognition

Factors Affecting This Stage and Negative Consequences
As mentioned earlier, pattern recognition is the process whereby the derived synthesized auditory memory percepts are compared to stored patterns in long-term memory, with perceptual identification and interpretation resulting from the best match. The ability to make the "correct" match is highly dependent on the accurate derivation of acoustic cues from the incoming stimulus and the extent to which the percepts have been stored accurately in long-term memory. Consequently, these processes are highly dependent on the same factors that have an impact on initial feature extraction, specifically the audibility of acoustic cues and temporal/frequency resolution.

In addition to acoustic cues, everyday discourse is rich in linguistic redundancy. The interrelationship of linguistic redundancy and speech intelligibility was first demonstrated by Miller, Heise, and Lichten (1950). Miller and associates assessed speech intelligibility for different speech materials in the presence of white noise. In one experiment, speech materials consisted of digits (numbers 1 to 9), sentences, and nonsense syllables. Miller and associates found that 50 percent intelligibility was reached at –14 dB S/N for digits (i.e., the overall speech level was 14 dB less intense than the noise signal presented), –4 dB S/N for words in sentences, and +3 dB S/N for nonsense words. Hence, the added redundancy allowed subjects to perform equally at poorer S/N ratios. In a second experiment, subjects listened to words presented in (1) isolation and (2) sentence context in the presence of background noise. The authors found that 50 percent intelligibility was reached at a 6 dB lower level when the words were heard in sentence context.

Boothroyd and Nittrouer (1988) examined the recognition of words at different S/N ratios (–15 to +10) using three types of sentences:

1. High predictability (i.e., grammatical sentences)
2. Low predictability (i.e., semantically anomalous)
3. Zero predictability (i.e., nonsense sentences)

The improvement in performance was quantified for the addition of both syntactic and semantic context. Boothroyd and Nittrouer found that the probability of word recognition in high-predictability sentences (i.e., both syntactic and semantic cues present) was 10 to 20 points higher than in low-predictability sentences (i.e., with only syntactic cues present) and 20 to 35 points higher than in zero-predictability sentences.

Knowledge of the topic of the sentence also aids speech perception. Garrett and St. Pierre (1980) examined subjects' ability to recall words in sentences presented at three different S/N ratios. These researchers found that subjects performed significantly better when the topic was given and that the gains derived were larger the poorer the S/N ratios.

These results strongly suggest that the ability to use linguistic and social context greatly facilitates spoken language perception, especially in noisy environments. Therefore, individuals who exhibit (1) an impoverished lexicon, (2) disorganized schema (such as those involving semantic relations), or (3) poor knowledge of syntactic rules will be negatively affected regarding the accuracy and speed to which they will be able to process spoken stimuli, and, in turn, in their ability to process incoming speech.

Recommended Management Strategies

In addition to the management strategies already recommended for addressing the negative consequences of feature extraction deficits, a number of strategies can be implemented to address deficits in pattern recognition. For example, for clients exhibiting a reduced lexicon, management techniques might include vocabulary building, semantic categorization (i.e., identifying categories to which items belong), and semantic mapping/associations (i.e., identifying attributes and functions associated with a particular item). Poor syntactic development can be addressed through one-on-one therapy or through commercially available programs. Pragmatic skills and social/world knowledge are often addressed through role-playing, simulated everyday activities, discussion, and computer software. The importance of all these strategies is to develop age-appropriate vocabulary and well-organized schema that allow for accurate and efficient processing and retrieval of information.

There are also number of compensatory strategies that may be extremely helpful. Because these individuals often require additional time to process information, they will benefit greatly from talkers using a somewhat slower rate of speaking (e.g., a newscaster's speech style) whenever possible. This technique allows them to keep pace with the conversation, especially if novel or complex topics are presented. Another extremely useful technique, especially for students or workers being trained on a new topic/skill, is for the individual to be informed of what new topics or vocabulary will be covered in upcoming lessons. This allows the individual to use the linguistic context to facilitate listening (i.e., top-down processing).

Short-Term Memory

Factors Affecting This Stage and Negative Consequences

The amount of information that can be held at any one point in short-term memory is contingent on three variables: (1) speed and accuracy to which incoming stimuli are processed, (2) speed and accuracy of retrieval of activated items from long-term memory, and (3) the length of time that items can be maintained in short-term memory. Deficits in any of these three abilities will decrease the individual's short-term memory span.

The speed and accuracy to which incoming items are processed has already been touched upon in the section on pattern recognition. A related skill is the efficiency to which items are retrieved from long-term memory. An example often mentioned in the computer literature may help to illustrate factors that can affect positively or negatively on the retrieval of items. This example concerns the manner in which files may be stored in computer memory. Files may be stored haphazardly—that is, without any clearly defined organization. For example, all of the files may be stored in one directory (e.g., one drawer of a file cabinet) without any discernible pattern that will allow for easy retrieval. When it comes time to locate this file, the individual may end up taking an inordinate amount of time before locating the desired file. On the other hand, if this same individual was to carefully plan a strategy for storing these files— for example, by categories and subcategories—the amount of time subsequently spent on retrieving them would be significantly reduced. In addition, computer files used most often by the individual would likely be the most easily accessed, since they would be the most salient in the individual's long-term memory. The importance of the computer analogy is to illustrate how prompt retrieval of items from long-term memory is highly dependent on the familiarity of items as well as the manner in which items have been stored in memory.

As mentioned earlier, Miller (1956) found that when item familiarity is low (such as word items of low-frequency occurrence), short-term memory span is reduced. This suggests that individuals having an impoverished lexicon may not be able to process and hold as much information in their short-term memory as their peers. If these same individuals were also to exhibit poorly disorganized schema and deficient knowledge of linguistic rules, they would likely need more time to process incoming information. In addition, they might not be able to use linguistic context to group the words into larger chunks.

As a result of these combined deficits, the individuals would likely process and retain fewer units of information per unit time, and the amount of information contained per unit would be less than that of their peers. These conclusions are supported by this author's work with students who are deaf. In those instances where students who are deaf exhibited language skills significantly below age peers, be it in sign or oral modality, they revealed a reduced short-term memory span, even when the task involved digit recall. When these same individuals were asked to recall sentences varying from 5 to 12 words in length, they tended to recall isolated words, many times out of sequence. (Interestingly, the number of words typically recalled by these students were identical to the number of digits that they recalled.) For these teens, the average number of digits/words recalled was on the order of 3 ± 1. Interestingly, this is the same number of units Miller (1956) found that adults typically recalled when presented with highly unfamiliar or nonsense words. Note that these students who were at age norms for language, be it oral or sign, did exhibit a short-term memory span within age norms.

The importance of rehearsal was discussed earlier in the context of the prominent role it plays in slowing the decay of items from short-term memory. Rehearsal comes into play when recalling numbers, writing down notes while in class, repeating directions to oneself, and so on. Individuals who do not have an adequate language base may not be able to effectively rehearse stimuli to themselves, and, as a result, exhibit a reduced short-term memory span. In fact, this may have contributed to the poor performance shown by many of the students who are deaf mentioned in the previous paragraph. It is also possible that many of these students had not acquired the necessary metacognitive skills required to do effective rehearsal.

Recommended Management Strategies

Management strategies to address deficits in short-term memory can be categorized by those addressing processing and retrieval versus the retention of items. A number of strategies addressing processing and retrieval of items have already been addressed under the topic of pattern recognition. However, one other strategy is noteworthy. When asked to respond to oral instructions, some individuals exhibit sequencing difficulty when repeating back information or in following instructions. There are many techniques that address sequencing difficulty, depending on the specific nature of the deficit. The following is an example of a technique that is often used to assist individuals who have difficulties in following directions. These clients are instructed to inform the communicator to provide one instruction at a time when *important* details/directions need to be absorbed. Clients are told to repeat each direction and then to summarize all of these directions at the end. This technique serves a number of purposes.

First, it allows the communicator to ascertain if and when a breakdown has actually occurred. Second, it allows for the communicator and the client to achieve success with less frustration. Last, this technique serves as a training tool that, hopefully, over time, will enable the client to follow a greater number of directions. A compensatory technique for those clients who can read and write is for the communicator, such as a teacher, to write down the directions or to have the client write down the directions personally. This last technique is often successfully employed with individuals suffering from memory decline.

Management strategies can be successfully employed as well in assisting individuals who have difficulty retaining items in short-term memory. Recall that the importance of rehearsal strategies is that they maintain and slow down the decay of items stored in working memory. Because rehearsal strategies are under an individual's conscious control, these skills can be readily taught. That is, rehearsal is a metacognitive skill whereby clients can be taught to think about the strategies they employ on a particular task. Rehearsal strategies include:

1. Memorization (i.e., item for item)
2. Mnemonic strategies (e.g., associating items by categories or a visual representation)
3. Grouping items into a smaller number of units (e.g., memorizing social security and telephone numbers)
4. Singing (e.g., learning the alphabet)
5. Elaborative rehearsal (e.g., reconstituting what has been heard for its most salient aspects rather than word for word)

In addition to formal techniques, there are a number of simple communications strategies one can use with individuals exhibiting a reduced short-term memory span. These include (1) informing the listener ahead of time to the topic of the discussion, (2) talking at a normal conversational speed but with frequent pauses to allow the individual to process the information in a relatively small number of chunks at any one point in time, and (3) restricting the use of nonfamiliar or complex terminology.

Attention

Factors Affecting This Stage and Negative Consequences

Attention involves the selection of strategies for processing certain stimuli in preference to others. To determine whether a deficit on a task is due to inadequate or inappropriate strategies rather than one of information overload, the clinician must first determine whether a client has developed the necessary skills for carrying out that particular task. For example, when a student listens to the teacher and takes notes at the same time, does that individual write down only the most salient details (hence, conserving attentional resources)? An initial assessment of the metacognitive aspects of these tasks allows the clinician to determine whether the problem is one of metacognition versus one of overload.

It should be clear to the reader that deficits in feature extraction, pattern recognition, and/or short-term memory will significantly affect an individual's ability to focus on a task. Individuals presenting with any of the preceding difficulties will expend significant energy to process information, even in a quiet setting. As long as the mental load is less than the residual capacity, these individuals will be able to process and recall the information. If competing stimuli were to be introduced into the environment, further energy would need to be expended toward the suppression of these irrelevant stimuli. For these individuals, this, in turn, could result in an inability to complete the task. Thus, the symptomatology in a difficult listening situation may suggest an attentive deficit when, in fact, the real difficulty may be due to an underlying deficit.

The relationship between load and capacity and its subsequent effects on attention can be examined as a function of different attention tasks. For example, the mental load entailed by a selective attention task can be systematically altered by changing the type of stimuli to be processed. On a selective attention task, one can vary the degree of difficulty by having the listener repeat single-syllable words versus sentences. Because the listener must expend more energy to process sentences, less residual capacity is available for suppressing the irrelevant, competing stimuli. If, in turn, this individual was then asked to attend to and recall paired sentences presented simultaneously to opposite ears (i.e., a divided attention task), the mental load would increase even further and could possibly approach or exceed residual capacity. Note that most adults have little or no difficulty on any of these tasks, whereas many individuals with learning disabilities do experience difficulties, especially on the divided attention task. This difficulty might be due to many of these individuals having less residual capacity and/or expending a significantly greater amount of mental energy when processing the target stimuli.

Although the term *attention deficit disorder* and the accompanying symptoms might suggest an attentional allocation problem, this author has found only one instance where this failure on a selective or divided attention task could be attributed purely to an attentional allocation deficit. In all other cases, these individuals exhibited deficits in either phonological and/or lexical decoding, sequencing, fading short-term memory, reduced short-term memory span, and so on. Interestingly, the literature in recent years (Barkley, 1989, 1991) indicates that most scientists no longer view attention deficit disorder with hyperactivy (ADHD) as an attention disorder but rather as a disorder of behavior regulation or of resource allocation (a processing orientation). That is, individuals with ADHD have an inability to use an appropriate behavioral repertoire in a particular setting. These findings suggest that if one is to ascertain the true auditory processing capabilities of individuals diagnosed with ADHD, one should do so when these individuals are on appropriate medication so that their behavior patterns do not interfere with the results.

Recommended Management Strategies

Management of attentional deficits can be grouped into two categories, depending on the nature of the deficit. The first involves management strategies for addressing deficits in metacognitive skills essential to the success of an attentional task. One such strategy is helping a client to ascertain the critical elements when listening to a presentation; for example, the listener may be placing equal emphasis on all of the components of speech rather than to those items pertinent to understanding the crucial ideas being conveyed. Another example might involve the listener who is experiencing listening difficulty in a multitalker situation; metacognitive strategies might include instructing the listener to focus on differentiating suprasegmental cues (such as pitch, rhythm, accent) specific to the target talker from the competing talkers.

The second category addresses deficits related to when the processing load exceeds the individual's reserve capacity. In all likelihood, these deficits are due to underlying deficits related to feature extraction, pattern recognition, or short-term memory and, therefore, entail management strategies specific to these breakdowns. In those instances where listening difficulties appear to be due to an attentional allocation deficit, as manifested by an inability to suppress irrelevant stimuli, a successful management strategy would be to increase the signal-to-noise ratio. This could be accomplished by instructing the client to (1) decrease the distance between the client and talker, (2) move away from the noise source, (3) attend to the talker's face (i.e., speechread), or (4) use an assistive listening device.

SUMMARY

In some ways, examining the memory and attention difficulties exhibited by a particular client is somewhat analogous to looking at the tip of an iceberg. What is seen may belie what is hidden underneath. Because each iceberg exhibits different characteristics, different solutions are required when working with individuals with memory and attention deficits. Yes, it may be true that the child is fidgeting in class, unable to stay on task, and has difficulty following directions, but the underlying causes for these difficulties may be different among individuals and the choice of management strategy will need to differ accordingly. That is, one cannot classify individuals by one term and use the same strategy for all individuals; in fact, this approach may be deleterious to some. Therefore, as stated in the onset of this chapter, if clinicians are to successfully address memory and attention deficits, they should be aware of the underlying memory and attention processes engaged in spoken language perception, be aware of the types of breakdowns that can occur, and be able to choose the appropriate strategies to address these deficits.

REFERENCES

Baddeley, A. D., Thomson, N., & Buchanan, M. (1975). Word length and the structure of short-term memory. *Journal of Verbal Learning and Verbal Behavior, 14,* 575–589.

Barkley, R. (1989). Attention deficit disorder with hyperactivity. In E. Mesah & L. Terdal (Eds.), *Behavioral assessment of childhood disorders* (pp. 69–104). New York: Guilford Press.

Barkley, R. (1991). Foreword. In L. Braswell & M. Bloomquist (Eds.), *Cognitive-behavioral therapy with ADHD children.* New York: Guilford.

Boothroyd, A., Erickson, F. N., & Medwetsky, L. (1994). The hearing aid input: A phonemic approach to assessing the spectral distribution of speech. *Ear & Hearing, 15,* 432–442.

Boothroyd, A., & Medwetsky, L. (1992). Spectral distribution of /s/ and the frequency response of hearing aids. *Ear and Hearing, 13,* 150–157.

Boothroyd, A., & Nittrouer, S. (1988). Mathematical treatment of context effects in phoneme and word recognition. *Journal of Acoustical Society of America, 84,* 101–114.

Broadbent, D. E. (1958). *Perception and communication.* Oxford: Pergamon.

Broadbent, D. E. (1984). The Maltese Cross: A new simplistic model for memory. *Behavioral and Brain Sciences, 7,* 55–94.

Brokx, J. P. L., and Nooteboom, S. G. (1982). Intonation and the perceptual separation of simultaneous voices. *Journal of Phonetics, 10,* 23–36.

Carhart, R., & Tillman, T. (1970). Interaction of competing speech signals with hearing losses. *Archives of Otolaryngology, 91,* 273–279.

Collier, R., & Hart, J. (1975). The role of intonation in speech perception. In A. Cohen & S. G. Nooteboom (Eds.), *Structure and process in speech perception* (pp. 107–121). Heidelberg: Springer Verlag.

Dorman, M. F. (1986). Temporal resolution, frequency selectivity, and the identification of speech. *The Hearing Journal, 3,* 24–26.

Elliott, L. L. (1982). Effects of noise on perception of speech by children and certain handicapped individuals. *Journal of Sound Vibration, 16,* 10–14.

Finitzo-Hieber, T., & Tillman, T. W. (1978). Room acoustic effects on monosyllabic word discrimination ability for normal and hearing-impaired children. *Journal of Speech and Hearing Research, 33,* 440–458.

Flexer, C., Millin, J. P., & Brown, L. (1990). Children with developmental disabilities: The effect of sound field amplification on word identification. *Language, Speech and Hearing Services in Schools, 21,* 177–182.

Garrett, R. L., & St. Pierre, L. (1980). Message comprehension as a function of intelligibility and advance knowledge of the topic. *Journal of Auditory Research, 22,* 71–80.

Gopher, D., & Donchin, E. (1986). Workload—An examination of the concept. In K. R. Boff, L. Kaufman, & J. P. Thomas (Eds.), *Handbook of perception and human performance.* New York: John Wiley and Sons.

Gregg, V. H. (1986). *Introduction to human memory.* London: Routledge and Kegan Paul.

Hawkins, D. (1984). Comparisons of speech recognition in noise by mildly-to-moderately hearing impaired children using hearing aids and FM systems. *Journal of Speech and Hearing Disorders, 50,* 132–141.

Hawkins, H., & Presson, J. (1986). Auditory information processing. In K. R. Boff, L. Kaufman, & J. P. Thomas (Eds.), *Handbook of perception and human performance. Volume II: Cognitive processes and performance.* New York: John Wiley and Sons.

Hirsh, I. J. (1950). The relation between localization and intelligibility. *Journal of Acoustical Society of America, 22,* 196–200.

Kahneman, D. (1973). *Attention and effort.* Englewood Cliffs, NJ: Prentice Hall.

Katz, J. & Harmon, C. (1982). *Phonemic synthesis: Blending sounds into words.* Allen, TX: Developmental Learning Materials (now available through Vancouver, Washington: Precision Acoustics).

Klatzky, R. L. (1984). *Memory and awareness: An information-processing perspective.* New York: W. H. Freeman.

Licklider, J. C. R. (1948). The influence of interaural phase relations upon the masking of speech by white noise. *Journal of Acoustical Society of America, 20,* 150–159.

Lindamood, C. H., & Lindamood, P. C. (1975). *Auditory discrimination in depth.* Allen, Tx: DLM Teaching Resources.

Massaro, D. W. (1970). Preperceptual auditory images. *Journal of Experimental Psychology, 85,* 411–417.

Massaro, D. W. (1972). Preperceptual images, processing time, and perceptual units in auditory perception. *Psychological Review, 79,* 124–125.

Massaro, D. W. (1975). *Experimental psychology and information processing.* Chicago: Rand McNally.

Massaro, D. W. (1976). Auditory information processing. In W. K. Estes (Ed.), *Handbook of learning and cognitive processes. Volume IV: Attention and memory* (pp. 275–320). Hillsdale, NJ: Lawrence Erlbaum.

Massaro, D. W., & Cohen, M. M. (1975). Preperceptual auditory storage in speech recognition. In A. Cohen & S. G. Nooteboom (Eds.), *Structure and process in speech perception* (pp. 226–243). Heidelberg: Springer Verlag.

Miller, G. A. (1956). The magical number seven, plus-or-minus two: Some limits in our capacity for processing information. *Psychological Review, 63,* 81–97.

Miller, G. A., Heise, G. A., & Lichten, W. (1950). The intelligibility of speech as a function of the context of the test materials. *Journal of Experimental Psychology, 41,* 329–335.

Norman, D. (1979). Perception, memory, and mental processes. In L. G. Nillson (Ed.), *Perspectives on memory research* (pp. 121–144). Hillsdale, NJ: Lawrence Erlbaum.

Pickett, J. M., Revoile, S. G., & Danaher, E. M. (1983). Speech cue measures of impaired hearing. *Hearing Research and Theory, 2,* 57–92.

Ross, M. (1986). Classroom amplification. In W. R. Hodgson (Ed.), *Hearing aid assessment and use in audiologic habilitation* (pp. 231–265). Baltimore: Williams and Wilkins.

Rumelhart, D. E., & Ortony, A. (1977). The representation of knowledge in memory. In H. C. Anderson, R. J. Spiro, & W. E. Montague (Eds.), *Schooling and the acquisition of knowledge.* Hillsdale, NJ: Lawrence Erlbaum.

Stark, R. E., & Tallal, P. (1979). Analysis of stop consonant production errors in developmentally dysphasic children. *Journal Acoustic Society of America, 66,* 1704–1712.

Tallal, P., Miller, S. L., Bedi, G., Byma, G., Wang, X., Nagarajan, S. S., Schreiner, C., Jenkins, W. M., & Merzenich, M. M. (1996). Language comprehension in language-learning impaired children improved with acoustically modified speech. *Science, 271,* 81–84.

Thorndyke, P. W. (1977). Cognitive structures in comprehension and memory of narrative discourse. *Cognitive Psychology, 9,* 77–110.

Tyler, R. S. (1988). Signal processing techniques to reduce the effects of impaired frequency resolution. *The Hearing Journal, 9,* 34–47.

Wingfield, A. (1975). The intonation-syntax interaction: Prosodic features in perceptual processing of sentences. In A. Cohen & S. G. Nooteboom (Eds.), *Structure and process in speech perception* (pp. 146–159). Heidelberg: Springer Verlag.

Wyer, Jr., R. S., & Srull, T. K. (1989). *Memory and cognition in its social context.* Hillsdale, NJ: Lawrence Erlbaum.

6

APPLICATION OF FM TECHNOLOGY TO THE MANAGEMENT OF CENTRAL AUDITORY PROCESSING DISORDERS

RAMONA L. STEIN
Nu-Ear Hearing Aid Center, Inc., Youngstown OH

Frequency modulated (FM) amplification systems have been used for years by children with hearing impairments to improve speech understanding in adverse classroom listening environments. These systems reduce the distance between the teacher and the student with a hearing impairment, which effectively overcomes the negative effects of background noise and reverberation. Peripheral hearing loss is one factor that can affect speech processing ability. Central auditory processing disorders (CAPD) also affect a child's ability to process a degraded, reduced, or distorted speech signal. Children with hearing impairments and those with CAPDs are both vulnerable to the adverse listening conditions found in the typical classroom. One solution to the less-than-optimal classroom listening environment is to fit the child with CAPDs with an FM amplification device.

FM amplification systems are wireless devices that receive distant auditory input, amplify, and then transmit that signal to the ear of a listener. A microphone connected to a transmitter and worn by the person speaking picks up the desired signal and converts it from an acoustic to an electrical signal. This electrical signal is transmitted via FM band waves to the receiver, where it is amplified by about 10 dB. Attached to the receiver are headphones that transform the electrical signal back into an acoustic signal, which is presented to the listener.

Factors such as background noise, a teacher's dialect or accent, and inconsistent vocal intensity of the teacher's voice can degrade the quality of the desired acoustic signal. The presence of a central auditory processing disorder further hinders the child's ability to fill in the missing or degraded portions of the acoustic signal and prevents accurate interpretation of the signal. FM amplification systems are designed to help overcome these problems by reducing the speaker-to-listener distance to approximately six inches, and improving the signal-to-noise (S/N) ratio by 8 to 12 dB. Thus, the learning environment can potentially be improved by providing a high-quality acoustic signal and reducing the effects of background noise and reverberation.

Because most classrooms are not good listening environments, FM systems are often recommended for classroom use subsequent to diagnosis of CAPD. Additionally, FM amplification systems have been recommended as an environmental modification for children with learning disabilities (Willeford & Billger, 1978). Improved attending behaviors such as eye contact with and body orientation toward the sound source have been documented with the use of FM auditory trainers by normal-hearing children with learning disabilities (Blake, Field, Foster, Platt, & Wertz, 1991). Few if any data-based studies have been conducted to evaluate the effectiveness of FM amplification with CAPD children. Positive anecdotal reports have been published regarding normal-hearing children with and without CAPDs in classrooms using group amplification systems (Allen, 1990; Berg, 1990). Classroom teachers and administrators have reportedly noted overall improvements in attentiveness and academic performance of all students in classrooms equipped with sound field FM systems.

However, systematic data-based research is needed to examine the effects of FM amplification devices on the academic performance of children diagnosed with CAPD. Such studies should qualify and quantify improvements in academic performance and classroom behavior subsequent to fitting a CAPD child with an amplification device. Further, benefits observed in non-CAPD children in classrooms fit with sound field amplification devices would assist school systems in justifying the purchase of these devices. Despite the lack of validation studies of this technique, FM amplification devices are currently being used in classrooms with CAPD children. This chapter will provide guidelines for use of FM amplification systems in CAPD children within the premise that more research needs to be conducted in this area.

FM amplification systems are one of many remediation techniques that are useful for children with CAPDs. FM amplification is not appropriate for every child diagnosed with CAPDs, nor should it be considered a "cure" for CAPDs. Just as a test battery approach is advocated for assessment of CAPDs, a similar approach should be considered when planning remediation activities. Although FM amplification is appropriate for many children with CAPD, alternative remediation techniques, such as noise desensitization training, should also be considered.

The following discussion presents a series of guidelines for selecting, fitting, and evaluating FM amplification systems used for remediation of CAPDs. Specific areas covered include which evaluation tools may be used as indicators of need for an FM amplification device, typical FM amplification systems recommended for children with CAPDs, variables to consider in the selection and fitting of FM units, follow-up procedures, techniques for evaluating the effectiveness of the FM system, educating support personnel, alternatives to FM technology, and the need for future research.

BENEFIT OF FM TECHNOLOGY IN CAPD MANAGEMENT

The personal FM units and sound field FM systems used with CAPD children provide mild amplification of desired signals, such as the teacher's voice, and reduces the distracting effects of background noise and reverberation by improving the S/N ratio in the classroom. Information obtained from parents and educators prior to the CAPDs evaluation may provide the audiologist with an indication of the potential benefits of FM technology. For example, parents or educators may note that the child is easily distracted from an auditory signal when trying to listen in the presence of competing noise, has difficulty understanding information presented auditorily, and frequently asks that questions and directions be repeated. These informal reports may lead the parents and teacher to request a more formal evaluation.

Questionnaires such as the Fisher Auditory Problems Checklist (Fisher, 1976) and the Children's Auditory Processing Performance Scale (Smoski, Brunt, & Tannahill, 1992) can be helpful prior to conducting a comprehensive CAPDs evaluation by providing a general idea of which tests to include in the battery. A comprehensive CAPDs evaluation should assess four main areas: temporal processing, processing of dichotic signals, auditory closure, and auditory figure-ground (Musiek & Chermak, 1994). Following diagnosis of CAPDs, a remediation plan should be designed according to the deficits found. This discussion is limited to remediation of specific deficits through use of FM amplification, but other therapeutic programs should be considered. A number of these programs are detailed elsewhere in this book. Several alternatives to FM amplification will also be briefly discussed.

Before considering whether FM amplification is suitable for a particular child, certain deficits must be present. Children exhibiting difficulties on tasks that involve binaural separation, binaural integration, auditory closure, and listening in the presence of competing background noise are possible candidates for FM devices. Even if a child demonstrates deficits in these areas on a CAPDs assessment, a corresponding improvement in listening while using an FM device may not occur. Therefore, it is crucial to proceed with a systematic subjective and objective evaluation to determine whether FM amplification is indeed helpful. This subjective and objective evaluation of FM amplification is detailed here. Table 6.1 lists several assessment tools that may be useful in determining the need for an FM device.

TYPES OF FM TECHNOLOGY

According to Sanders (1965), average noise levels measured in occupied classrooms range from 55 to 65 dB(A). Blair (1977) measured S/N ratios of +3 dB in regular classrooms. For children with sensorineural hearing loss, the average ambient noise levels for unoccupied classrooms should not exceed 30 to 35 dB(A), and the S/N ratio should be greater than +15 dB for optimal speech perception (American Speech-Language-Hearing

TABLE 6.1   Tests That May Indicate Need for FM System

Test	Skill Tested
SSW	Binaural integration
SCAN subtests:	
Auditory figure ground	Auditory figure ground
Filtered words	Auditory closure
Dichotic digits	Binaural integration
SSI-ICM	Auditory figure ground
SSI-CCM	Binaural separation
Time-compressed speech	Auditory closure

Association, 1994). Since no such published standards exist for normal-hearing children, it has been recommended that the standards for children with sensorineural hearing loss should be applied to children with normal hearing (Crandell & Smaldino, 1995). In regular classrooms, maintaining a 30 to 35 dB(A) ambient noise level and a +15 dB S/N ratio is not practical. Yet, it is possible to attain the recommended standards in most classrooms through use of either personal or sound field FM amplification systems. Personal FM devices worn by normal-hearing children with CAPDs provide mild (10 to 15 dB) amplification of the teacher's voice and are designed for use by one child at a time. Sound field FM systems are designed to provide mild amplification of the teacher's voice through loudspeakers, and thus all children in a particular class can benefit.

The audiologist recommending either a personal or a sound field FM system will be faced with a variety of factors when making recommendations to school administrators regarding the purchase of these systems. The decision to fit a child with a personal FM unit, or to equip the child's classroom with a sound field FM system, depends on the number of children in the same classroom exhibiting similar listening problems. In many cases, it is more cost effective for the school to invest in a sound-field system than several personal devices. Another factor to consider is the child's grade level. A personal device may be more appropriate for a child who changes classes several times during the school day. A personal device may also be more appropriate if the child will be attending one-to-one therapy or tutoring sessions.

Personal FM Systems

Personal FM units consist of a transmitter, which is worn by the classroom teacher, and a receiver, which is worn by the student (see Figure 6.1). Most personal FM systems offer several microphone options for transmitters and several listening options for receivers. For example, the Phonic Ear Easy Listener transmitter can be coupled with an omni-directional or directional microphone clipped either to the teacher's clothing or worn on a lavalier cord. Other options include a boom microphone worn on a headset or a conference microphone. The boom microphone offers the most freedom of movement for the teacher and the most consistent acoustic signal, because the distance from the microphone to the teacher's mouth remains constant. The conference microphone may be useful in smaller classrooms or during group work and group discussions.

The personal FM receiver can deliver the amplified acoustic signal to the listener in a number of ways. The audiologist may select a Walkman-style headset, monaural or binaural earbuds, a stetoclip, or a teleloop

FIGURE 6.1   Easy Listener PE300 Personal FM System (educational version) with Transmitter (on shelf), Directional Microphone, Receiver, and Headset

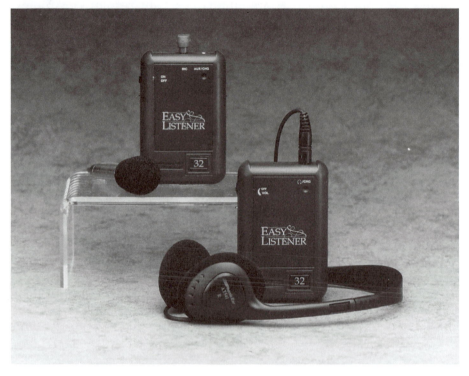

Photo courtesy of Phonic Ear Inc. © 1997 Phonic Ear Inc.

coupled with a personal hearing aid. The Phonic Ear Easy Listener offers both a standard and an attenuated Walkman-style headset.

Sound Field FM Systems

Sound field FM systems generally consist of a transmitter, a receiver, and up to four loudspeakers (see Figure 6.2). These systems amplify the desired acoustic signal 10 to 12 dB above the level of the ambient classroom noise. As with the personal FM system, a number of options are available. Microphone options for the Phonic Ear Easy Listener transmitter include a lavalier-style directional microphone or a boom microphone worn on the head. The receiver includes a variety of controls that

FIGURE 6.2   **Easy Listener Sound Field System (with four speakers)**

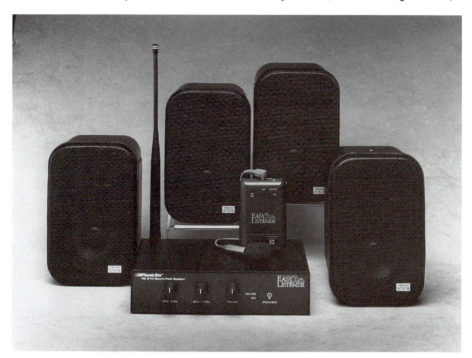

Photo courtesy of Phonic Ear Inc. © 1997 Phonic Ear Inc.

the audiologist may adjust according to the needs of the students in a particular classroom. For example, the sound level of the FM signal as well as that of an auxiliary input can be controlled. Also, a tone control allows for adjustment of the frequency response for a variety of listeners and listening environments. The loudspeakers may be permanently mounted or placed on shelves or floor stands so they can be rearranged easily.

SELECTION AND FITTING OF FM UNITS: VARIABLES TO CONSIDER

When recommending an FM amplification system, it is important to be specific. The audiologist should recommend the most appropriate device based on a prefitting assessment of the child's needs. This preliminary information may be helpful to demonstrate need for the FM amplification system to school administrators. Another method for demonstrating need and usefulness of the FM device is to simulate a noisy classroom environment for teachers and administrators. Presenting cassette recordings of noise or having a television or radio playing in the background while demonstrating the FM device will allow individuals who are inexperienced with the device to assess the benefits firsthand.

The preliminary assessment should include a classroom observation by the audiologist and a functional listening evaluation. The functional listening evaluation targets the child's listening abilities in an environment intended to be similar to a typical classroom (DeConde Johnson, Benson, & Seaton, 1997). This evaluation can be completed with or without the FM device. A comparison of the results of this evaluation with and without the device can be useful to demonstrate benefit provided by the device. SPIN sentences, PSI sentences, PB-K words or WIPI words are some of the materials suggested for use with this evaluation. The child's language skills should be considered prior to selecting evaluation materials. Eight lists are presented, with easy conditions at the beginning and end, and more difficult conditions in between.

Conditions that are varied are close/distant, noise/quiet, and auditory/auditory visual. In the close condition, the noise source and the examiner are 3 feet in front of the student. In the distant condition, the noise source is 3 feet in front of the student and the examiner is 15 feet in front of the student. In the quiet condition, the student hears the examiner's voice at a level of 75 dB(A) measured 1 foot from the examiner's mouth. In the noise condition, the background noise measured at the student's ear should average 60 dB(A). In the auditory-only condition, the student receives no visual cues from the examiner. In the auditory-visual condition, the examiner presents the sentences using auditory and visual information. A sample presentation protocol is shown in Table 6.2. The entire evaluation using sentence material takes 30 minutes (DeConde Johnson, Benson, & Seaton, 1997).

When recommending an FM system, the audiologist should clearly state the purpose of the device and whether a personal or sound field device is being requested. If the child has an individualized education plan (IEP), provisions for the FM amplification system should be included. The IEP must specify when the child is to wear the device during the school day. FM amplification devices purchased by the school district are, in most cases, only for use at the school during school hours. If an arrangement cannot be made between the school and the parent regarding use of the FM device outside of school hours, the parents may wish to consider purchasing a second system themselves.

TABLE 6.2 Sample Presentation Protocol for the Functional Listening Evaluation as Described by DeConde Johnson and von Almen

Auditory/Visual	Close/Distant	Quiet/Noise
1. Auditory/visual	Close	Quiet
2. Auditory	Close	Quiet
3. Auditory/visual	Close	Noise
4. Auditory	Close	Noise
5. Auditory/visual	Distant	Noise
6. Auditory	Distant	Noise
7. Auditory	Distant	Quiet
8. Auditory/visual	Distant	Quiet

Note: This order places the easier tasks at the beginning and end of the evaluation.

EVALUATING THE EFFECTIVENESS OF THE FITTING

The selection and fitting of all types of amplification devices must be approached systematically to ensure maximum benefit to the wearer. The audiologist should evaluate the effectiveness of FM amplification devices using both objective and subjective measures.

Objective Measures

Thibodeau and Saucedo (1991) reported high variability in the electroacoustic performance of similar models of FM amplification systems. Although based on the use of FM systems by children with hearing impairments, certain recommendations made by these authors are applicable to FM devices worn by children with CAPDs. Specifically, a comprehensive evaluation of FM amplification systems is recommended. This evaluation should include an electroacoustic analysis of the FM receiver, headphones, and microphone. Since no standards exist for the use of FM amplification by individuals with normal hearing, use of the guidelines for individuals with hearing impairments has been recommended. These guidelines specify a semi-annual evaluation of FM devices worn by children. The evaluation may include coupler measurements, real ear measurements, questionnaires, and classroom observations (American Speech-Language-Hearing Association, 1994). Real ear measurement is often substituted for coupler or electroacoustic measures for Walkman-style headphones and earbuds due to coupler problems.

Sound field testing may be used to determine whether the FM unit improves the child's speech intelligibility in background noise. The evaluation is generally conducted in a sound room using a message-in-competition task (Stach, Loiselle, Jerger, Mintz, & Taylor, 1987). The child is seated with one speaker facing and one speaker behind him or her. Sentences are presented through the speaker facing the child at a fixed level in the range of 40 to 60 dB SPL, and single-talker discourse is presented through the speaker behind the child using message-to-competition ratios (MCR) ranging from +20 to –30 dB. The transmitter's microphone is placed eight inches in front of the speaker facing the child during the evaluation. Repeated measures are taken with 10 sentences presented at each MCR. A percent correct score is calculated for each MCR (Stach et al., 1987). Using this method, it is possible to assess and document the benefit a CAPD child obtains through use of a personal FM amplification system.

Subjective Measures

The audiologist fitting the FM system should maintain involvement after the device has been fit. Classroom observations should be conducted pre- and postfitting by the audiologist and teacher. Consultation with the classroom teacher is very important to ensure that the device is worn and used properly by both the student and the teacher. The audiologist's and teacher's observations of the child postfitting are valuable, but the best indicator of a successful fit is the child's willingness to continue wearing the unit. In determining the suitability of an FM amplification system, it is helpful, but not mandatory, that the audiologist and the teacher notice an improvement in listening and attending. More important evidence of a successful fit is the child's willingness to wear the device. If the child rejects the device or shows little or no sign of improvement in listening behaviors, alternative training may be needed. This training may be used in place of an FM amplification system, or in addition to the system.

EDUCATING SUPPORT PERSONNEL

A national long-term study indicates that audiologists play a relatively small role in the selection, maintenance, and troubleshooting of FM amplification devices worn in school by children with hearing impairments (Maxon, Brackett, & van den Berg, 1991). Further, the authors noted a trend toward less involvement on the part of audiologists over the five years during which two separate groups of respondents were sampled. Another important finding of this study is that children with hearing impairments received orientation and training sessions for their FM devices from FM manufacturers, rather than from an audiologist.

Since most audiologists are not employed by school systems, support persons often are enlisted to monitor children fit with personal FM amplification. Due to their diverse and heavy caseloads, those audiologists that are employed by the schools will most likely need additional help from others to monitor the FM devices. Possible participants in a monitoring program for FM amplification devices include speech-language pathologists, classroom teachers, and teacher's aides. Responsibilities can range from performing an electroacoustic analysis of the device to making sure the device is charged on a daily basis.

To be successful, all CAPDs remediation programs depend on active participation on the part of the child, parents, and teachers. The cooperation of administrators and the understanding of classmates is also necessary. Administrators, parents, and educators need to know how the FM device works in order to evaluate improvement. Teachers and parents, if applicable, must be trained to monitor the FM systems daily. A brief daily visual and listening check can ensure that the systems are operating adequately (Ross, 1992). The child with CAPDs, as well as classmates, can also assume some responsibility for monitoring the FM device. The child with CAPDs should be trained to use the system and to inform the teacher when the system is malfunctioning. Other responsibilities for the child with CAPDs may include recharging the battery, transporting or storing the system, and reminding the teacher to turn on the transmitter.

A brief in-service presentation should be offered by the audiologist fitting the FM system. Topics to cover include basic information about CAPD, classroom acoustics, and FM amplification systems. Some educators may be familiar with FM amplification systems through prior exposure to students with hearing impairments. During the in-service presentation, the audiologist should highlight the differences between use of FM devices by children with hearing impairments and those with normal hearing. Students should be instructed to use only their assigned FM unit (Thibodeau & Saucedo, 1991). This recommendation is especially important considering most children with CAPDs fit with FM amplification have normal hearing. Borrowing an FM unit that was intended to be worn by a child with a hearing impairment could be both uncomfortable and harmful. Teachers and other school personnel must be informed that microphones and headphones should not be interchanged between devices. It is valuable if the audiologist maintains contact with and is available for periodic consultation by school personnel.

ALTERNATIVES TO FM TECHNOLOGY

The benefits of using an FM device may be immediate and dramatic. The child may be more attentive, able to follow directions with improved accuracy, require fewer repetitions, show an increase in classroom participation, and even show overall academic improvement. It is important to remember that these effects are evident only while the child wears the FM device. Table 6.3 lists a few of the approaches that may be helpful to a child who demonstrates difficulty listening in the typical classroom setting. These procedures may be used in place of or in addition to the use of an FM amplification system. The approaches listed include noise desensitization training, auditory closure activities, phonemic synthesis training, phonemic analysis training, and use of compensatory strategies. The advantage of these approaches over the FM device is that they can provide the CAPD child with a more permanent solution to adverse listening conditions. On the other hand, the benefits of the FM device are realized only while it is being worn. Other methods can be found in other chapters of this book.

NEED FOR FUTURE RESEARCH

Although FM amplification is often recommended after CAPDs have been diagnosed, a trial period with a device is essential prior to the purchase of the equipment. Although many children can benefit from the improved S/N ratio provided by an FM amplification system, improvements in listening behaviors and academic performance are not guaran-

TABLE 6.3 Additional/Alternative Approaches to the Use of an FM Amplification System

Approach	Goal
Noise desensitization training	Improve speech understanding in noise.
Auditory closure tasks	Improve ability to comprehend speech when it is distorted in some way.
Phonemic synthesis	Improve decoding of speech signal. Improve listening skills.
Phonemic analysis	Improve listening skills.
Compensatory strategies	Improve assertive listening behaviors.

teed. Some children may benefit more from therapy activities than from the use of an FM device. Some children may refuse to wear, or wear improperly, an FM device. Some parents and classroom teachers may not be committed to the use of an FM device, thus reducing the child's opportunities for successful use of the device.

SUMMARY

This chapter has outlined a systematic approach to the use of FM amplification systems as one possible remediation tool for children diagnosed with certain central auditory processing deficits. Although the use of FM amplification devices by children with CAPDs is increasing, a number of questions remain unanswered. More research is needed in order to improve the use of FM amplification as a remediation technique for children with CAPDs. The following list of questions is the product of issues raised in this chapter, and is by no means all-inclusive.

1. Does the use of personal FM units or sound field amplification improve the academic performance of children diagnosed with CAPDs?
2. If sound field FM amplification does improve the academic performance of children diagnosed with CAPDs, is the degree of improvement comparable to that observed in non-CAPD students from the same classroom?
3. Is one particular CAPDs test a better indicator of potential benefit from use of FM amplification?
4. Is FM amplification an adequate replacement for various remediation techniques (e.g., noise desensitization therapy)?

REFERENCES

Allen, L. (1990). WHAT? Speaker system helps in the classroom. *Educational Audiology Newsletter, 3,* 7.

American Speech-Language-Hearing Association. (1994). *Standard on acoustics in classrooms.*

Berg, F. (1990). Recent research on sound field FM. *Educational Audiology Newsletter, 1,* 6.

Blair, J. (1977). Effects of amplification, speechreading, and classroom environment on reception of speech. *Volta Rev, 79,* 443–449.

Blake, R., Field, B., Foster, C., Platt, F., & Wertz, P. (1991). Effect of FM auditory trainers on attending behaviors of learning-disabled children. *Lang Speech Hear Serv Sch, 22,* 111–114.

Crandell, C. C., & Smaldino, J. J. (1995). Classroom acoustics. In R. J. Roeser & M. P. Downs (Eds.), *Auditory disorders in school children* (3rd ed.) (pp. 219–234). New York: Thieme Medical Publishers.

DeConde Johnson, C., Benson, P., & Seaton, J. (1997). *Educational audiology handbook*. San Diego: Singular Publishing Group.

Fisher, L. I. (1976). *Fisher Auditory Problems Checklist*. Cedar Rapids, IA: Grant Woods Education Agency.

Maxon, A. B., Brackett, D., & van den Berg, S. A. (1991). Classroom amplification use: A national long-term study. *Lang Speech Hear Serv Sch, 22,* 242–253.

Musiek, F. E., & Chermak, G. D. (1994). Three commonly asked questions about central auditory processing disorder: Assessment. *Am J Audiol,* 23–27.

Ross, M. (1992). *FM auditory training systems.*

Sanders, D. (1965). Noise conditions in normal school classrooms. *Except Child, 31,* 344–353.

Smoski, W. J., Brunt, M. A., & Tannahill, J. C. (1992). Listening characteristics of children with central auditory processing disorders. *Lang Speech Hear Serv Sch, 23,* 145–152.

Stach, B. A., Loiselle, L. H., Jerger, J. F., Mintz, S. L., & Taylor, C. D. (1987). Clinical experience with personal FM assistive listening devices. *The Hearing Journal, 5,* 1–6.

Thibodeau, L. M., & Saucedo, K. A. (1991). Consistency of electroacoustic characteristics across components of FM systems. *J Speech Hear Res, 34,* 628–635.

Willeford, J. A., & Billger, J. M. (1978). Auditory perception in children with learning disabilities. In J. Katz (Ed.), *Handbook of clinical audiology* (pp. 410–425). Baltimore: Williams & Wilkins.

7

THE M³ MODEL FOR TREATING CENTRAL AUDITORY PROCESSING DISORDERS

JEANANE M. FERRE
Audiologist, Private Practice

The auditory perceptual therapy model described in this chapter is predicated on the hypothesis that, although differing in site of dysfunction, some auditory perceptual deficits due to central disorder are characterized by communicative, educational, and psychosocial manifestations similar to those due to peripheral auditory dysfunction. Early site-of-lesion research in the area of CAPDs included patients presenting with complaints typical of hearing impairment but found to have normal or near normal peripheral hearing sensitivity. That research established that for patients with demonstrable central auditory nervous system (CANS) disorder, a reduction of intrinsic redundancy was created that resulted in listening/hearing difficulties not unlike those created at the periphery by conductive and/or sensorineural hearing loss. By logical extension, patients presented with similar behavioral and/or diagnostic profiles have been presumed to be suffering from a similar loss or inefficiency within the CANS, even in the absence of demonstrable neurological disorder.

This body of work, as well as neuropsychological research, provide compelling evidence that a wide range of auditory skills are subserved by specific and identifiable regions within the CANS. Further, disorders among these skills are likely the result of dysfunction in one or more of these regions. In fact, in its recent report, the ASHA Task Force on Central

Auditory Processing (ASHA, 1995) defined *central auditory processing disorder* as observed deficiency/deficiencies in sound localization and/or lateralization, auditory discrimination, auditory pattern recognition, recognition of degraded acoustic signals, recognition of competing acoustic signals, or the processing of temporal aspects of auditory signals. That document went on to describe the ways and means by which basic neuroscience supports this model of CAPD.

What remains less well defined is the exact relationship between and among central auditory processing abilities and educational, communicative, and psychosocial behavior. Anecdotal reports spanning several decades, as well as correlational data show low to moderate, but still significant, correlations between and among tests and skills. These reports and data offer strong support to the assertion that educational success, communicative proficiency, and/or psychosocial wellness are dependent, at least in part, on the adequacy of central auditory skills and the integrity and efficiency of the CANS (Myklebust, 1954; Kaluger & Kolson, 1969; Protti, Young, & Bryne, 1980; Rampp, 1980; Flowers, 1983; Ferre, 1992).

More recent neurophysiological research provides the clearest and most promising findings to date to support these assertions. Specifically, the identification of the mismatch negativity or MMN evoked response and the later occurring P300 response. The MMN, believed to reflect the automatic, preattentive processing of fine acoustic differences of speech, appears to be a correlate of speech perception (see Naatanen & Kraus, 1995, for comprehensive review). The P300, generated by several multisensory cortical and subcortical structures, may be providing a measure of cognitive integration of auditory discrimination (Picton, Woods, Baribeau-Braun, & Healy, 1977).

When used in concert, clinical audiological CAP measures and evoked response study become powerful tools in the diagnostic process. They give evidence that within the heterogeneous population labeled CAPD, there exists a subgroup of clients/patients with identifiable perceptual disorder, the cause of which appears to be inefficient ability to decode fine acoustic differences in speech signals.

Called *auditory decoding deficit,* the diagnostic profile includes poor performance on tests of degraded speech and speech-in-noise, with the right ear often poorer than the left. (Ferre, 1992; Bellis & Ferre, 1996). CAP test errors tend to be phonemically similar to the target, and retention, discrimination, and sound blending skills are often weak. Sequelae include poor academic performance in spelling and reading and/or speech-language deficits in the areas of vocabulary, syntax, and semantics.

The marked similarities between this profile and that of the patient with peripheral involvement are clear. In fact, initial referral for these patients is typically standard audiologic evaluation to assess hearing sensitivity. Thus, it would follow that management strategies effective for use with patients having peripheral involvement should also be effective with patients presenting with CAPD—the nature of which is specific auditory decoding deficit.

As suggested by ASHA (1995), one of the goals of the CAP assessment process is an intervention program designed to improve everyday function and life satisfaction for clients/patients. That report categorized various CAPD interventions into two broad approaches, one directed toward enhancing the client's own resources and a second directed toward enhancing the auditory signal and improving the listening environment. Similarly, a recent Educational Audiology Association newsletter (1996) featuring CAPD describes CAPD management as falling into one of three approaches: direct therapies to improve listening skills or noise sensitivity, strategies for coping and problem solving, or environmental modifications.

Several recent reports related to CAPD management make clear the need for a cohesive and comprehensive management philosophy that recognizes the interactions that may exist between and among central auditory abilities and communication, education, and/or behavior, and therefore utilizes strategies and techniques from all three approaches (Bellis, 1996; Bellis & Ferre, 1996; Chermak, 1996).

Like a table that has three legs and needs all three to stand, it is clear that the only effective management for CAPD must include (1) modification of the client's environment to minimize auditory overload and maximize coping, (2) use by the client *and* the teaching of compensatory and coping strategies, and (3) direct therapeutic techniques designed to improve the deficient auditory (and/or other related) skills. To do less denies the known complexity of the system with which one is dealing and flies in the face of known success of the similar philosophy employed with patients having peripheral hearing loss. Thus, this model is fundamentally traditional aural rehabilitation implemented, with some modifications, for patients presenting with what may be thought of as nontraditional or central hearing loss (Myklebust, 1954).

ENVIRONMENTAL MODIFICATIONS AND COMPENSATORY TECHNIQUES

For clients diagnosed with specific auditory decoding deficit, recommendations covering environmental modification and clients' use of compensatory strategies include, but may not be limited to, the following items:

1. Preferential classroom seating wherein line of vision to the primarys-peaker is emphasized over distance.
2. Reduction of extraneous noise, including the use of sound-absorbing materials in the classroom or home, rearrangement of furniture, or monitored use of high-quality noise-reducing earplugs such as the ER-15 or ER-20 styles.
3. Use of repetition *only* if it will enhance the acoustic clarity of the signal or the use of repetition with an associated visual cue. Although simple repetition allows the listener access to cues that may have been missed initially, a poorly perceived signal may remain such even after several repetitions if these are of poor acoustic quality. This model's preference for children with perceptual disorder is the use of rephrasing to provide a new, perhaps better-perceived, target having additional linguistic redundancy.
4. Use of attention-getting devices such as calling child's name or using "tag" words to mark key points (e.g., *first, last, before, after, this, that,* etc.).
5. Provision of instructions, information, written and verbal assignments, and the use of a classroom "buddy" as needed for clarification.
6. Use of clear, concise, explicit language when asking questions or giving instructions.
7. Reduction, elimination, and/or modification of oral examinations.
8. Waiver of secondary or collegiate foreign language requirement or, in lieu thereof, American Sign Language (ASL) courses. Many states recognize ASL for foreign language credit at secondary and/or collegiate levels (NICD, 1996).
9. Use of assistive technology or services, including, high-quality tape recorder, computer, personal or, soundfield FM units, books on tape, notetakers, and so on.

Since many of these patients, particularly children, may exhibit significant psychosocial, academic, and/or speech-language sequelae, the direct therapy aspect of this plan includes recommendation for additional evaluation and/or treatment for disordered receptive/expressive language, reading, spelling, writing, self-image, and/or peer relations. Like the transdisciplinary approach used in diagnosis, the total management of CAPD must likewise be a team effort, including speech-language pathologists, audiologists, psychologists, neuropsychologists, educational specialists, and so on, as needed.

The key component of this management plan's direct therapy leg is the inclusion of specific goals that can be accomplished over a relatively short time span that are designed to improve the client's ability:

1. To perceive speech
2. To tolerate the adverse effects of extraneous noise
3. To use visual information to enhance understanding
4. To use metalinguistic/metacognitive strategies for improved communication
5. To understand and use assistive technology
6. To advocate for self in the communication situation

The reader is referred to Chapter 4 in this book for a comprehensive treatment of metacognitive/metalinguistic management strategies and to Chapter 6 for a discussion of the use of assistive technology, particularly FM systems, for management of CAPDs.

AUDITORY-VISUAL TRAINING THE M³ WAY

In this therapy, any communication event is characterized as the combined interaction of three key elements—the message, the medium, and me—hence, M³ model. *Message* refers to quality and characteristics of the signal, *medium* refers to quality of the listening environment, and *me* refers to those attitudes, strategies, and skills that the listener brings to the listening situation.

The therapy sessions use a combination of consultation/information giving, role-playing, drill work, and games to accomplish the objectives associated with each goal. Throughout the therapy sessions, using the methods just described, the client will learn how negative changes in any one component of the communication triad will adversely affect communication and, conversely, how positive changes can enhance the experience.

Key issues to be addressed related to the *message* include:

1. Familiarity, acoustic and linguistic
2. Extrinsic redundancy, acoustic and linguistic
3. Method of presentation (e.g., closed or open set)
4. Availability of nonauditory cues (e.g., visual)

With respect to the *medium*, or listening environment, four other topics are discussed:

1. Distance
2. Lighting
3. Reverberation
4. Noise

For the *me* component, the key concepts are:

1. Listener's physical wellness
2. Listening attitude and behavior
3. Visualization
4. Self-help

Speech Perception Improvement

Specific activities designed to improve the client's, particularly a child's, speech perception skills are likely to be familiar to many audiologists and speech-language pathologists. In this model, tasks requiring auditory or auditory-linguistic closure are included along with phoneme training. Sloan's (1995) phoneme training program is utilized, with modification, in which students must accurately discriminate minimally paired consonant, CV and/or VC pairs. In addition, M^3 clients must also discriminate minimally contrasted vowels, such as short e and short i (*beg* versus *big*) or short e and long a, (*wet* versus *wait*) and accomplish all tasks both in quiet and in a background of equal loudness competing noise.

Auditory closure activities for clients with decoding deficit include games in which the child will *complete the rhyme* with and without specific clues to the target. The following are samples of each task:

With Specific Clue

Therapist: Fill-in the word that rhymes (sounds like) for each of the following. All the rhyming words are colors.

The new blanket on my bed, is a bright shade of _____.

We searched up and down for my shoes that are _____.

Without Specific Clue

Therapist: Finish the rhyme; it could be any word at all.

From my bed I awoke when I smelled _____.

You know all about Jack and Jill—they're the ones who went up the _____.

Another rhyming game requires the child to generate rhymes for randomly selected target words using an *alphabet line*. In this activity, all speech sounds, excluding vowels, are written in a line form. The child draws a card from the therapy deck and must make rhymes of the target word using the available targets. The initial step in this activity is the use of a die or other number indicator to determine the number of rhyming words required. After repeated success with a finite number of targets, the child comes "off the dice" and must make rhymes using *all* available initial sounds or sound blends. Points are given only for real English words, excluding proper names. Slang usage is allowed. These restrictions provide opportunity for the therapist to build vocabulary by immediately discussing those words for which the child may have received a point but was not aware of the word's meaning. Similarly, by having the child read the words on each card, speech-to-print skills are enhanced along with basic sight vocabulary, particularly for words having irregular spellings (e.g., *nest* and *guest*). In addition to enhancing sound-blending skills, the activity can improve general sequencing and organization skills as the child is encouraged to start at the beginning, work in order, and try every possibility.

Alternative methods for children who have difficulty, reading the targets (i.e., those with very weak sound-symbol, association) include the following:

1. The therapist provides the new initial sound as a prompt and the child provides the word (e.g, for the word *cat* and the target *str*, the therapist provides *str* and the child produces *strat*).
2. The therapist provides all components of the target in discrete segments and the child blends the sounds (e.g., therapist: *str - a - t;* child: *strat*). This is similar to the task requirements of the Phonemic Synthesis Test (Katz, 1983).

Finally, for those children unable to accomplish the tasks using auditory or auditory and visual cues, tactile cues and instruction are provided. One such child would "mark" the initial phoneme with the right hand and the VC "final" portion with the left hand. By physically closing the hands together, smooth sound blending was accomplished (e.g., left hand: *k;* right hand: *at;* as hands were brought together, the child produced *cat*).

Noise Tolerance and Auditory Training

Auditory-only and auditory-visual activities are adapted from Garstecki's Auditory-Visual Training Paradigm (1981). In the paradigm, four parameters are manipulated, one at a time, over a preset range from high redundancy to low redundancy. The four parameters are type of signal, type of background noise, signal-to-noise ratio (S/N), and type of available visual cue. In addition, in the M³ model, two other variables are added: number of target repetitions and message format.

For auditory-only conditions, therapy objectives are:

1. To recognize everyday sentences presented in the soundfield without repetition in a background of ipsilateral multispeaker babble at a –10 S/N with 95 percent accuracy.
2. To recognize single-syllable words presented in the soundfield without repetition in a background of ipsilateral multispeaker babble at a –5 S/N with 85 percent accuracy.

For auditory-visual (A-V) conditions, objectives are:

1. To recognize everyday sentences presented with lipreading cues (A-V presentation) in the soundfield in a background of ipsilateral multispeaker babble at a –20 S/N with 75 percent accuracy.
2. To recognize single-syllable words presented with lip reading cues in ipsilateral multispeaker babble at a –10 S/N ratio with 80 percent accuracy.

For both auditory-only and A-V conditions, sentences must be repeated exactly as stated to be counted as correct. Paraphrasing, although discussed and encouraged as a legitimate communication strategy, is not counted toward total percent correct. By allowing paraphrasing as a strategy, though, the therapist may gain insights into the child's expressive language/memory-based skills. In one such case, a client demonstrated after several months of therapy markedly improved ability to tolerate excessive extraneous noise by repeating every word of each sentence presented. However, the child's consistent reporting of those words, grossly out of order, even in the absence of interfering noise, suggested deficiency in output/sequencing skills. In this case, a severe output-expressive deficit was masked by significant receptive disorder and did not become apparent until after substantial remediation of the auditory decoding and associated receptive language problems.

Use of Visual Cues

Visual-only training in this therapy includes discussion/instruction in the use of body language, gestures, pictures, symbols, and punctuation marks (e.g., the communicative meaning of *?* or *!*). A state's *Rules of the Road* manual is an excellent therapy tool to teach children how pictures alone can contain significant messages (contact your Secretary of State's office for copies). As noted previously, the use of printed words is included in an effort to expand basic sight vocabulary.

In addition, each client receives formal speech reading/lip reading training beginning with the ability to discriminate visual sameness/difference. The therapy then proceeds through a discussion of the visual characteristics of speech sounds grouped and ranked according to difficulty to lip read. Therapy games consist of both identification of compound words from among a closed set of printed words or pictures and, depending on the client's age, identification of sentences from among a closed set. For the latter drills, natural English sentences generated by the therapist and client or synthetic sentences from the Synthetic Sentence Identification (SSI) (Jerger & Jerger, 1974) serve as targets. Although third-order approximations of English syntax, Jerger's synthetic sentences are more difficult to perceive auditorily than natural English sentences due to their reduced linguistic redundancy. Interestingly, an examination of clients' performance have suggested that they may be somewhat easier to perceive visually, possibly for the same reason.

Metalinguistic Strategies and Assistive Technology

Woven throughout therapy activities are examples and pointers designed to enhance the client's use of metalinguistic strategies for improved communication. Use of both high-predictability and low-predicatibility sentences help frame a discussion of how contextual and situational cues may be used to assist understanding. Word association, categorization, and labeling games are included throughout to encourage discussion of the various styles and strategies that listeners employ to manage auditory-verbal information. As mentioned previously, paraphrasing, organizational strategies, and vocabulary building are included throughout the sessions. Also discussed are the use of verbal rehearsal, information chunking, and mnemonics to aid understanding, retention, and recall of auditorily presented material.

Designed to improve the signal-to-noise ratio reaching the ear, assistive listening devices (ALDs) have been used in the management of CAPD. However, not all children with CAPDs can be expected to benefit from ALD use. Based on their diagnostic profile, children with specific auditory decoding deficits appear to be most likely candidates for successful ALD use, especially personal FM systems. For these children, poor performance in noise may be related not to simple distractibility but rather to the underlying inefficiency of the discrimination skills. As a result of the masking effect noise has on speech targets, extrinsic redundancy is reduced, thus overloading an already inefficient system. Unlike traditional amplification where the speech signal and any ambient noise may both be amplified (even with noise suppression circuitry), the physical configuration of the personal ALD has the effect of *pulling the target signal away from the noise* via mild gain amplification, thereby pushing the noise further into the perceptual background. This results in a significantly more favorable S/N ratio and, in turn, improved speech reception/perception.

It cannot be emphasized enough that a diagnosis of CAPD does not, in and of itself, mean a recommendation for an ALD. Further, the client, parents, and other service-delivery personnel (e.g., classroom teacher) must receive sufficient consultation and training in device usage, advantages, disadvantages, trouble-shooting, and so on. When used with proper diagnosis and monitoring, personal assistive listening devices have shown promise in improving auditory attention, short-term memory, and auditory discrimination and perception (Shapiro & Mistal, 1985, 1986; Stach, Loiselle, Jerger, Mintz, & Taylor, 1987; Blake, Field, Foster, Plott, & Wertz, 1991).

For one such child, the device created a dramatic positive change, not only in classroom listening but also in overall speech perception. After a three-month hiatus from aural rehabilitation, during which the child wore a personal FM system daily in school, the child's ability to recognize degraded speech was found to be 27 percent better than scores for similar measures obtained six months earlier. Although neuromaturation and the brief therapy in which the child participated contributed to this improvement, it is unlikely that these were the sole explanations. It is possible that device usage in this case not only improved speech recognition during the periods of actual use but it also provided a sufficiently stable, high-quality signal over time as to improve overall efficiency of auditory discrimination skills.

Self-Advocacy

It is essential that any management plan for the client with CAPD include training in and/or discussion of those skills that will empower the client. Assertiveness training, situational problem solving, and self-help tips all should be included in order to build the client's confidence in his or her own skills and coping strategies. Even with very young children, the therapist must be honest about the client's strengths and weaknesses and the rationale for therapy. In addition, therapy success will be affected by the attitudes of and follow-up by the client's significant others.

Self-advocacy activities should have the following objectives:

1. The client will understand the nature and manifestations of the CAPD.

2. The client will demonstrate ability to improve the communication event through alteration of his or her own behavior.
3. The client will demonstrate ability to improve the communication event through alteration of the environment.
4. The client will demonstrate ability to improve the communication event through alteration of the message.
5. The client will demonstrate ability to enlist others to assist in improving the communication event.

Two examples of improved self-advocacy are provided here. A child had been described by teachers as impolite and immature based on persistent use of the word *huh* when repetition was needed. At a parent-teacher conference just four weeks after therapy had begun (and without the teacher's knowledge that therapy was in progress), the teacher reported to the mother that the child had become a very mature, well-mannered child. What was the child's new strategy? Instead of "Huh" to get information repeated, a switch was made to "I'm sorry, I didn't hear that last (first) part. Could you repeat that, please?" Interestingly, a recent report of adult hearing-impaired listeners found that the listeners had greater success consistently obtaining repetition of information when stating, "I have a hearing loss, what did you say?" as opposed to the simple request for repetition of "What did you say?" (Martin & Ross, 1994).

Another child demonstrated improved self-help during the fifth therapy visit. At that visit, the child was found seated in the therapist's chair located against a far wall as opposed to the client's chair located directly between two speakers from which background noise emanated. When questioned, the child reported, "Today, I'm going to sit here, because it's too noisy over there and I can't hear you. This is better for me."

GAUGING SUCCESS

The therapist relies on a combination of measures in determining treatment efficacy. Comparison of pre- and posttherapy assessments, observation, parent reports, classroom notes, teacher checklists, and extent to which specific behavioral objectives are met are all useful in determining whether the overall management plan has been effective. In addition, though, electrophysiological data may be a useful tool in assessing treatment success. As neurophysiological research has indicated, lack of stimulation to the CANS, for whatever reason, may result in identifiable loss of system integrity as measured by evoked potentials. The use of direct therapy techniques in the management of CAPD is based on the assumption that the converse is true—increased stimulation will enhance functional integrity.

This being the case, pre- and posttherapy evoked potentials studies may provide useful insights regarding the combined effects of neuromaturation and benefit derived from therapy. For one client, pretherapy evoked potentials indicated absent MMNs across a wide range of contrasts. These results were consistent with behavioral diagnosis of specific auditory perceptual (decoding) deficit. Therapy outcome measures following 20 one-hour therapy sessions suggested that fine discrimination had improved but remained somewhat deficient for the child's age. Evoked potential study at approximately the same time revealed presence of a misshaped MMN for several contrasts and persistent absence for several others. Following another course of therapy, behavioral results suggested age-appropriate auditory discrimination while evoked potentials study revealed present and well-formed MMN responses for all but the most difficult contrasts tested. The child was dismissed from therapy, and recent reevaluation of CAP skills revealed no evidence of significant CAPDs. Recent evoked potentials study revealed well-formed normal responses for all stimuli, ABR through the P300.

This one case, as well as the several others mentioned, are not sufficient empirical evidence to prove this model's efficacy. However, these cases illustrate the following:

1. Direct intervention can improve central auditory perceptual skills for at least some clients.
2. There is an immediate need for treatment-specific outcome data related to CAPDs.
3. Behavioral and electrophysiological techniques must be "married" not only for diagnostic purposes but also for obtaining efficacy data.
4. The overall success of any CAPDs management plan depends as much on the effectiveness of the specific strategies employed as it does on the professionals' understanding of basic principles of assessment and rehabilitation and the underlying neuroscience upon which those principles are based.

REFERENCES

American Speech-Language-Hearing Association. (1995). *Central auditory processing: current status of research and implications for clinical practice. A report from the ASHA Task Force of central auditory processing.* Rockville, MD: Author.
Bellis, T. J. (1996). *Assessment and management of central auditory processing disorder in the educational setting.* San Diego, CA: Singular Publishing Group.

Bellis, T. J., & Ferre, J. M. (1996). Assessment and management of CAPD in children. *Educational Audiology Monograph, 4,* 23–27.

Blake, R., Field, B., Foster, C., Plott, F., & Wertz, P. (1991). Effect of FM auditory trainers on attending behaviors of learning-disabled children. *Language, Speech and Hearing Services in the School, 22,* 111–114.

Chermak, G. (1996). CAPD: Management—A comprehensive approach to managing central auditory processing disorders. *EAA Newsletter, 1,* 12.

Educational Audiology Association. (1996, Spring). *CAPD: Three approaches to remediation,* Tampa, FL: Author.

Ferre, J. (1992, November). *CAT files: Improving the clinical utility of central auditory function tests.* Paper presented at the American-Speech-Language-Hearing Association Annual Convention, San Antonio, TX.

Flowers, A. (1983). Auditory perception, speech, language & learning. Dearborn, MI: Perceptual Learning Systems.

Garstecki, D. (1981). Auditory-Visual Training Paradigm for hearing-impaired adults. *Journal of the Academy of Rehabilitative Audiology, 14,* 223–238.

Jerger, J., & Jerger, S. (1974). Auditory findings in brainstem disorders. *Arch Otolaryngol, 99,* 342–349.

Kaluger, G., & Kolson, C. (1969). *Reading and learning disabilities.* New York: Grune & Stratton.

Katz, J. (1983). Phonemic synthesis. In E. Lasky & J. Katz (Eds.), *Central auditory processing disorders: Problems of speech, language and learning* (pp. 269–295). Baltimore: University Park Press.

Martin, B., & Ross, M. (1994). The effect of repetition requests on the intensity of talkers' speech. *American Journal of Audiology, 3,* 69–72.

Myklebust, H. (1954). *Auditory disorders in children.* New York: Grune & Stratton.

Naatanen, R., & Kraus, N. (Eds.). (1995). Mismatch negativity as an index for central auditory function. *Ear and Hearing, 16,* 1–146.

National Information Center on Deafness (NICD). (1996, June). *States that recognize American Sign Language as a foreign language.* Gallaudet University, Washington, DC: Author.

Picton, T., Woods, D., Baribeau-Braun, J., & Healy, T. (1977). Evoked potential audiometry. *Journal of Otolarngology, 6,* 90–119.

Protti, E., Young, M., & Bryne, P. (1980). The evaluation of a child with auditory perceptual deficiencies: An interdisciplinary approach. *Seminars in Speech, Language and Hearing, 1,* 167–180.

Rampp, D. (1980). Auditory perceptual disorders: Speech and language considerations. *Seminars in Speech, Language and Hearing, 1,* 117–126.

Shapiro, A., & Mistal, G. (1985). ITE-aid auditory training for reading and spelling-disabled children: Clinical case studies. *Hearing Journal, 38,* 26–31.

Shapiro, A., & Mistal, G. (1986). ITE-aid auditory training for reading and spelling-disabled children: A longitudinal study of matched groups. *Hearing Journal, 39,* 14–16.

Sloan, C. (1995). *Treating auditory processing difficulties in children.* San Diego, CA: Singular Publishing Group.

Stach, B., Loiselle, L., Jerger, J., Mintz, S., & Taylor, C. (1987, May). Clinical experience with personal FM assistive listening devices. *Hearing Journal,* 24–30.

8

SPEECH AND LANGUAGE MANAGEMENT OF CENTRAL AUDITORY PROCESSING DISORDERS

M. GAY MASTERS
State University of New York at Buffalo

Children with central auditory processing disorders (CAPD) and language learning difficulties (LLD) have diverse management needs, necessitating the use of both remediation and intervention strategies. This chapter describes management techniques for three of the four types of CAPD disorder according to the Buffalo Model. The Buffalo Model describes over 10 years of attempts to identify the interaction between CAPD, LLD, and academic difficulties, and has been a major determinant of management needs and priorities. The audiological testing determines the category, or profile, of CAPD. The management techniques have been derived from the programs developed to ameliorate the noted deficiencies. These programs have been developed at the University at Buffalo Speech, Language and Hearing Clinic, including the five years of the Intensive Language Intervention Program (ILIP). ILIP is a model program for CAPD and LLD intervention services during summer recess from public school services.

MANAGEMENT PRIORITIES

The four categories of the Buffalo Model are: decoding, tolerance-fading memory, integration, and organization. These categories are fully described in Chapter 1 of this book. Individuals with CAPD often have characteristics of more than one profile under the Buffalo Model. We have found that it is most productive to begin addressing decoding needs as a first priority, followed by tolerance-fading memory needs. Management intervention for organization is typically implemented within the academic and home environments before or during the introduction of remediation techniques in the clinic. At present, we have developed no special techniques for use with those individuals with integration difficulties, but we have generally found it most beneficial to the individual when decoding therapies have been emphasized. The management programs for all children, and indeed for all individuals, with CAPD and LLD, should include self-awareness of the individual's needs as well as self-advocacy for receiving needed services. In all cases, management strategies are designed to reduce, eliminate, or compensate for the language, academic, and social interaction difficulties experienced by the child. In some instances, management strategies may be implemented for the child whose history places him or her at risk for these difficulties.

In this chapter, remediation strategies (i.e., therapy designed to alleviate the problem) are discussed first, followed by intervention (i.e., supportive and/or compensatory) strategies, for the three primary categories of the Buffalo Model: decoding, tolerance-fading memory, and organization. Initial strategies address skills that appear to be the basis for later skills. The clinician may choose to begin with the simplest skills and work through the hierarchy, or the clinician may probe to see how the child performs on a specific task and work upward from that level. However, it has been our experience that some skills that are present appear to be splinter skills. When we are at a more difficult level in the hierarchy and the child is unsuccessful for long periods of time, we move to the beginning of the hierarchy. Often, we find that the child lacks one or more of the skills at the bottom of the hierarchy.

PRESCHOOL MANAGEMENT

Many clinicians are aware of preschool children who have characteristics that suggest that they are at risk for later identification of a central auditory processing disorder. Typically, these children are known to have receptive and expressive language and speech disorders. We are particularly concerned about those children who demonstrate word-finding difficulties, cluttering disorders, and/or poor recall of repetitive, rote memory rhymes such as the ABC song, finger-plays (e.g., Five Little Monkeys), and nursery rhymes. The histories of school-age children with identified CAPD often show that these skills were poorly developed or absent when they were preschoolers. These skills are significant indicators of later literacy (Catts, 1991; Schuele, 1994). Many of the remediation techniques presented in this chapter, which are at the early stages of the hierarchy, can be utilized with those preschool children who are judged to be at risk for CAPD. These techniques are compatible with preschool curricula as well as the receptive and expressive language needs for these children.

DECODING

Individuals who experience difficulty with decoding aspects of central auditory processing have difficulty analyzing auditory information. Often, this difficulty appears to be with temporal aspects of the auditory information. That is, the individual responds after a delay and/or requests repetition of information, as if he or she did not have sufficient time to decode the message. The audiologist diagnoses this type of CAPD according to certain response patterns on simple linguistic units. Speech-language pathologists may gather complementary information using longer chunks of auditory information, such as phrases, sentences, and multistep directions in their language testing.

Remediation of decoding difficulties is aimed at improving the individual's efficiency with the processing of auditory information. Over the past 10 years, we have developed a hierarchy of therapy for decoding. Therapy may begin at the level of difficulty for the child. However, caution is suggested. It has been our experience that some individuals are able to perform tasks at the mid-level of the hierarchy, but are unable to perform those tasks that are thought to be easier, earlier steps in the hierarchy. We often recognize this discrepancy only after individuals experience failure at a higher level.

The decoding hierarchy begins with the ability to parse, or separate, language into sentences, phrases, and words, and ends with the metalinguistic ability to manipulate at the phoneme level. Syllable segmentation is a mid-level auditory skill in which the child is asked to recognize how many syllables are present in a word. However, the same skill of syllable segmentation becomes linguistically complex when the child is required to recognize the semantic effect of syllabic morphemes that affect meaning: prefixes and suffixes. Remediation activities include parsing into these units, as well as synthesizing these units back into wholes. These steps are described in the subsequent sections.

Parsing, or segmenting, the auditory stream into individual linguistic components begins soon after birth. The language style used by infant caregivers, termed *motherese*, appears to assist the child in recognizing these linguistic components, and aids in the development of semantics (Gleason, 1993). In motherese, the speaker speaks slowly and highlights significant words. This pattern of linguistic highlighting carries over to the rhythmical pattern and repetition of children's finger-plays (O-PEN SHUT them, O-PEN SHUT them, give a lit-tle CLAP), nursery rhymes, and much of preschool literature. Nursery rhymes and preschool books further highlight auditory patterns such as rhymes by placing the rhyming word in the final position of phrases. Auditory information is frequently repeated in preschool literature. Examples include Brown and Hurd's (1975) *Goodnight Moon* ("Goodnight bears and goodnight chairs... goodnight noises everywhere"), and Martin and Carle's (1992) *Brown Bear, Brown Bear, What Do You See?* ("Brown bear, brown bear, what do you see, I see a blue horse looking at me").

Thus, remediation at the most basic stage of decoding management targets the child's ability to separate chunks into sentences and words. Later, we ask the child to separate into the smaller segments, identifying the phonemes in words, and creating words from phonemes. We have seen only a limited number of children who are apparently unable to parse at the sentence or phrase level. These children are the ones who produce nursery rhymes or sing songs, but individual words cannot be identified. Often, the rhyme or song is recognized by the rhythm or tune, rather than by the words. With these children, tape recorders with loop-delay tapes and "slow and easy speech" lessons facilitate the child's ability to break down these memorized language forms into phrases. Once the child is at a phrase level, the focus turns to the word level.

Pretesting and remediation at the earliest stages of decoding involve segmentation, or parsing, at the phrase level. The child should be able to participate in group activities that involve finger-plays, nursery rhymes, and taking turns during the reading of a popular story. Therapy may focus on these activities first at the individual level but should move into group situations. It is crucial that the child be able to demonstrate the skills in a variety of situations with several different adults. Contexts include a separate room or corner of a room, or at home, with the speech-pathologist, parent, and teacher, as well as classroom aides and volunteers. Many catalogs for speech-language therapy materials include sources for literature with repetitive and predictable phrases. We have also found parallels to this level of CAPD therapy in the activities described for developing emergent literacy skills (Schuele, 1994).

Once the clinician is satisfied that the child is parsing at the phrase level, remediation begins to focus on more discrete and more metalinguistic aspects of the speech signal. Such analysis moves from words in isolation to identification and manipulation of individual speech sounds. This ability to manipulate sounds has been directly linked to reading ability (Catts, 1991; Swank & Catts, 1994). Commercial programs, computer software, and clinician-generated activities are available for this level of remediation.

Recognition and generation of rhymes, such as the Soundabet Game developed by Jeanne Ferre and discussed in Chapter 7 of this book, is an example of word-level manipulation. *Bailey's Book House* (Edmark Corporation, 1995) is a computer software program that contains an activity that requires the child to select the picture to complete a common nursery rhyme. At the easiest stage, all of the choices rhyme, as in *Rub a dub dub, three kids in a (tub, sub, shrub, club)*. A more complex task requires the child to choose from four choices, perhaps *tub, bell, cart, pie*. *Reader Rabbit 2* (The Learning Company, 1993) also targets rhyming in the game "Match Patch." Most phonics workbooks provide activities for rhyme identification and generation as a pre-cursor to reading. These workbook pages are ideal for therapy sessions or for involving parents in the child's therapy program.

Parsing at the word level is taught in a variety of ways, including cloze (or fill-in the blank) tasks, discrimination tasks, and rhyming. Cloze tasks can include typical collocations (word associations) such as *bread & butter,* as well as targets that are syntactically, semantically, or visually predictable: *You eat with a (spoon/fork)*. Once the child is demonstrating a familiarity with an interest in rhymes, cloze tasks can include rhymes as well: *That's my cup, said the _____ (pup)*. We have found Dr. Seuss books useful both to screen for this rhyming ability and to use as a therapy tool. Discrimination tasks can now be used to introduce more discrete auditory analysis skills. Minimal pairs of a semantic (e.g., *hairbrush, toothbrush, toothpaste*) or phonological (e.g., *k, cave, cage, cape*) nature can be used. The ability to produce rhymes spontaneously is a key indicator of the child's mastery of single-word parsing. For children 5 years or older, it is appropriate to include metalinguistic awareness by having the child indicate whether a particular rhyme is or is not a word. That is, the child who is creating rhymes from the initial target *hat* is asked to judge whether *gat* is a word.

Decoding remediation as described thus far is primarily contextualized, with visual and linguistic support minimizing the auditory attention and skill required. Syllable and phonemic segmentation and/or synthesis, however, place a heavy demand on the auditory system. Our experience has been that children who have little difficulty with syllabic and phonemic segmentation and synthesis are good auditory decoders. Success at this level is also a strong predictor of reading ability (Catts, 1991; Swank & Catts, 1994).

Syllable segmentation activities are appropriate for older preschool children. Visual support (e.g., a block per syllable) or motor accompaniment (e.g., tapping on a table or clapping) are used when working on syllable segmentation. Pictures of items with multisyllabic names can be used for marking and then cutting into the appropriate number of syllables. For example, *alligator* receives three lines across the picture and is then cut into four pieces, which may be manipulated like puzzle pieces. When a syllable is also a root word, such as *tooth + brush = toothbrush,* these puzzle pieces can be used for a more complex metalinguistic task, creating new words and judging whether they are actually words. For older children, it is a very useful activity, as language arts in school includes work on hyphenation and/or prefix/suffix by about grade 4. In the clinic, syllable segmentation work may be more developmentally acceptable for older children by working on prefix/suffix and hyphenation of curriculum vocabulary, rather than tapping out syllables on the table.

Phonemic parsing and synthesis is the final step in the therapy hierarchy currently in use at the State University of New York at Buffalo Clinic. Almost any phonics workbook can be adapted for decoding remediation, and several commercial programs are available for this stage. *Auditory Discrimination in Depth* (Lindamood & Lindamood, 1975) is a parsing program, and *Phonemic Synthesis* (Katz & Fletcher, 1982) is an example of a synthesis approach to phonemic level decoding.

Remediation utilizes a slow speaking rate with frequent repetition of key words or phrases. By repeating key words or phrases at the end of a sentence, the child's ability to parse the language stream into sentences, phrases, and words is facilitated. For example, children with a CAP decoding profile will benefit from pairing actions to pertinent words (e.g., finger-plays such as Itsy Bitsy Spider or Five Little Monkeys), exaggerated intonation, and extension of familiar sentence frames to classroom activities. For example, new vocabulary may be introduced by modifying the popular *Brown Bear* (Martin & Carle, 1992) phrase: "Caitlin, Caitlin, what do you see? I see the fire engine looking at me."

Intervention for individuals with a decoding CAPD is aimed at managing the environment so that there is as little stress on the individual's processing skills as possible. Visual support, either in picture format or print, is used whenever possible to supplement auditory information. An example of picture format at the preschool level is the classroom job chart, with a depiction of both the task (e.g., line leader) and the child assigned to the task. At the elementary school level, the daily routine is depicted in words and symbols on the chalkboard or on the child's desk. Beginning at the middle school level, the child is provided with an outline of the class lesson; overhead projectors may be used in addition to the chalkboard for the teacher to write pertinent notes while lecturing.

Curricula that teach auditory attention are valuable intervention tools. *Listening to the World* (Goldman & Lynch, 1980), a curriculum program appropriate for early elementary school children, focuses on auditory attention and memory. Classroom teams may also create their own approaches that emphasize listening skills. Children are rewarded for good listening through stickers, points, or simply the opportunity to participate in enjoyable auditory activities. Off-task behavior is not punished or commented on, except through the omission of the reward.

To aid a child with a CAP decoding problem, the teacher may be asked to make teaching modifications. For example, the teacher may be asked to slow down his or her speaking rate, at least for critical information. The teacher may also need to repeat instructions and information, and obtain the individual's attention by touch, eye contact, or physical proximity. Physical proximity also serves to improve the signal-to-noise ratio, which seems to improve decoding ability.

TOLERANCE-FADING MEMORY

Individuals with a tolerance-fading memory CAPD typically show impulsivity and forgetfulness in response to auditory information, as well as sensitivity to noisy backgrounds. An individual with a tolerance-fading memory disorder has difficulty in completing multiple-step instructions (e.g., "Get the box and kiss the bear") or multiple-attribute directions (e.g., "Get the *large, blue box* on the *second* shelf"). Difficulty may include missing portions of the directions or completing directions in an incorrect order. At times, it appears that the individual misses a portion of the direction because of premature or impulsive responding, while at other times, it appears that the individual has forgotten a step at the beginning or middle of the direction.

Remediation and intervention for tolerance-fading memory difficulties encompass two basic premises: Improve the individual's ability to remember multistep or multiattribute information and improve the individual's ability to perform in background noise. The first premise, improving auditory memory, involves the use of compensatory intervention strategies as well as remediation practice that may improve auditory memory span. The second premise, improving performance in background noise, is also known as *noise desensitization,* and involves cognitive awareness of noise, its affect on the individual's performance, and practice in various types of noise. For both premises, the individual is encouraged to develop the ability to advocate for himself or herself in a variety of situations. We suggest stressing functional activities over repetition of arbitrary word lists and digit recall.

Functional activities are drawn from or mimic the individual's activities of daily living. Classroom routines and lessons as well as household chores provide opportunities for tolerance-fading memory therapy. A client may practice repeating telephone numbers, locker combinations, directions to a friend's house, or specific math problems assigned for homework. In the State University of New York at Buffalo Clinic, scavenger hunts direct children to the vending machine area, where they report which soda is under the second button, and which candy bar is located under E-7, and how much money is required to purchase these items.

Auditory memory is enhanced by the use of several different techniques, including rehearsal, chunking, imagery, and notetaking. In our experience, auditory memory therapy needs to be more individualistic than the clearly hierarchical decoding progression. Techniques that we have found beneficial are briefly discussed here. Chapter 5 of this book also includes additional information to aid those with auditory memory problems.

Rehearsal is an extremely useful technique for helping the individual remember auditory information, and one that most of the general population uses automatically. It is almost second nature for an individual to repeat a telephone number or list of items to buy at the grocery store. However, individuals with CAPD may have one of two problems with rehearsal. Many of the children we see in our clinic, ranging from preschoolers to middle school children, do not use rehearsal at all. An almost equal number of children use this strategy, but in an immature manner. This immature manner is often problematic in the classroom. In this case, *immature* refers to those children who repeat instructions verbatim—rather than repeating only key information—and/or at a volume that is conversational level or louder. The verbatim information approach can be ineffective, as the child may miss a direction while repeating. Typically, children are disruptive if the information is repeated at conversational level in the classroom.

Both types of children, nonrehearsers and immature rehearsers, benefit from a sequential approach to rehearsal. Verbatim repetition is replaced by isolation and repetition of key elements. Once the individual is able to repeat the key elements, practice involves reducing volume until the repetition is through lip movement, or subvocal rehearsal, only. Finally, the individual replaces subvocal rehearsal with "words in your head"—silent rehearsal. During this practice in rehearsal, additional compensatory strategies such as chunking, imagery, and notetaking can be added.

Chunking is the organization of material into fewer bits of information. Chunking requires a metalinguistic skill, in that the items must be grouped, or "chunked," into logical segments, typically using categories. These segments are learned, one at a time, until the whole list is memorized. Thus, a child may learn a 20-item grocery list, presented aloud, once the chunks of "fruits," "meats," and "breads" are highlighted.

A hierarchical sequence for imagery in auditory memory therapy is easily implemented. Therapy materials are commercially available, including excellent lessons in the *Listening to the World* (Goldman & Lynch, 1980) program, and functional multistep directions may be created using items in the individual's environment. The individual is encouraged to "mark" the items (e.g., doll, book, and candle from a set of six items), first by physically touching and then by using eyes only. Typically, the individual also verbally repeats the items while using imagery assistance. The goal of imagery therapy is mental pictures, associated with quiet rehearsal.

Props are also used for multistep directions. The use of multistep directions often reveals the interaction of poor decoding skills on faulty auditory memory, particularly when unusual directions are given. For example, a student clinician in our clinic recently designed a following-directions activity using four scenes (a tree, a hill, a lake, and the sky) and a variety of animals. The instructions were to "Put the (animal) in/on/under the (scene)," and included directions that did not make sense, such as "Put the marine animals in the sky." The client routinely omitted the second step of the three-step directions. The clinician would repeat the directions, allowing the child to check her work. During the repetition, when the child no longer needed to focus on the first and last steps, it became clear that she had never processed the middle step. On repetition, the child responded, "Put the octopus in the tree? That's silly!" for the second direction, in the same fashion as she had commented on unusual directions in the first or second step. It appeared that decoding and auditory memory interacted to prevent this middle step from being processed; she was able to retain and respond (process) the first and last step but did not appear to "hear" the second step at all.

Notetaking is a useful compensatory strategy for poor auditory memory, and an important life skill. Children can learn the power of note-taking from the common childhood game of Picnic ("I'm going on a picnic and I'm taking X, Y, and Z"). Children often automatically point to the person who first included a particular item as an aid in recall. For those children who have sound-symbol association, they record the first letter of the item or use a chart of the alphabet to aid in memory. Thus, they learn how written notes, in conjunction with repetition, can result in the recall of a list of 26 or more items. Taking notes requires that an individual recognize key details and be able to rephrase information. Individuals highlight key points in a text as it is read aloud, then later fill in the blanks on a prepared sheet from a lecture. Finally, rephrasing from a lecture is taught.

Noise desensitization therapy is critical in the treatment of a tolerance-fading memory CAPD. For individuals with this type of disorder, noise can exacerbate the effect of auditory memory and decoding difficulties. In addition, for some individuals, noise can cause physical symptoms such as headaches, stomach aches, fatigue, and/or irritability. Our experience has been that children are often unaware of how performance and physical well-being are affected by different kinds of noise. The impact of noise on a particular individual is especially important for the school-age child, who spends approximately six hours a day in an environment with multiple sources of noise. At times, then, an important step in therapy is to identify how ability changes in noise, and to link certain physical symptoms with noise. Once the individual is aware of the effect of noise, controlled practice in various kinds of noise is provided. At the same time, the individual is given compensatory strategies to use in noisy environments, such as personal amplification devices, preferential seating, and ear plugs. See Chapters 6 and 12 in this book for additional information.

Noise desensitization therapy should follow some careful guidelines. For a young child, we feel it is important that noise therapy be conducted in the initial or middle portion of a therapy session. For those children who experience physical symptoms in addition to increased processing load in noise, the risk is present that the child will leave therapy in an irritable or ill state, and therefore have bad associations to the therapy session.

Noise is introduced at a low volume, selected by the child, using material that is at a level at which the child has demonstrated near 100 percent success in quiet. New vocabulary, new curriculum information, or recently established therapy goals (e.g., three-step directions) should be reserved for sessions at the end of the noise therapy hierarchy.

The noise hierarchy typically begins with white noise and ends with the type of noise that is most problematic for the individual. The clinician should include the type of noise present in the individual's environment; a site visit or noise checklist should be a component of this remediation step. We have had one case in which a child was unaffected by multitalker babble but experienced significant breakdown in discrimination ability and irritability with a low-volume buzz, similar to the noise produced by a loud fluorescent light or older radiator. Instrumental music, music with lyrics, radio or television programs, and school noise (e.g., classroom, gym, cafeteria) are used routinely in our clinic.

ORGANIZATION

Individuals with an organization profile of CAPD demonstrate poor auditory sequencing on audiological testing, and typically have poor sequencing in discourse. Retelling of stories is haphazard in terms of structure, such as beginning, middle, and end. Individual utterances may also show poor organization, as measured by excessive amounts of mazes (e.g., nonverbal fillers, repeated words and/or phrases), frequent pauses, and abandoned utterances. The organization type of CAPD often occurs in conjunction with decoding and/or tolerance-fading memory difficulties. Remediation techniques focus on metalinguistic and meta-cognitive development, such as detailed in Chapters 4 and 12 in this book.

Remediation of discourse difficulties is helpful in the management of the organizational aspects of a CAPD. Typical needs include topic initiation and maintenance, reduction of linguistic mazes, and clear sequence of events. A focus on narratives using story grammar (Johnston, 1982) provides a useful starting point for discourse therapy. Story grammar aids in the clarity of discourse by providing a logical and sequential structure. Individuals learn to introduce characters, time, and location of a narrative in the setting statements. The statement of a problem and the solution of the problem provide the maintenance of topic. Topic closure is facilitated through the formal ending present in story grammar.

Discourse therapy progresses through oral narratives into written language. Personal narratives are easiest, then children move to the retelling of their favorite stories, and finally to telling about a recently seen movie. Written language, either provided to the child (Norris, 1994), such as a favorite book, or produced by the child can assist in developing organized language.

As children enter the middle grades of elementary school, descriptions and persuasion/arguments are encountered in the curriculum. It is at this point in CAPD management that we introduce lessons on text structure and the production of written language. Different kinds of written language, or texts, contain different key words (Nelson, 1993) and are also structured differently. For instance, a description is different than a compare/contrast text. Recognition of words and structure in written text and auditory lectures can help the organizational abilities of the individual with CAPD. Pehrsson and Denner (1994) provide information on text structure and implications for development of reading and writing skills.

SUMMARY

This chapter has provided a brief overview of the complex management issues for individuals with CAPD. Remediation and intervention suggestions for decoding, tolerance-fading memory, and organizational central auditory processing difficulties were discussed. These suggestions were derived from over 10 years of collaboration between the audiologists and speech-language pathologists on staff at the State University of New York at Buffalo Speech, Language and Hearing Clinic. Our experience has indicated that management is most successful when comprehensive speech and language testing, in conjunction with school information, is integrated with audiological diagnosis. The individual is encouraged to fully participate in the management process and to take responsibility for requesting needed accommodations within his or her environment. Remediation appears to be most successful when decoding needs are emphasized over tolerance-fading memory and organization needs.

REFERENCES

Brown, M. W., & Hurd, C. (1975). *Goodnight moon.* New York: Harper Trophy.

Catts, H. W. (1991). Facilitating phonological awareness: Role of speech-language pathologists. *Language, Speech & Hearing Services in Schools, 22,* 196–203.

Edmark Corporation. (1995). *Bailey's book house.* Redmond, WA: Author.

Gleason, J. (1993). *The development of language* (3rd ed.). New York: Macmillan.

Goldman, R., & Lynch, M. E. (1980). *Listening to the world.* Circle Pines, MN: American Guidance Service.

Johnston, J. R. (1982). Narratives: A new look at communication problems in older language-disordered children. *Language, Speech and Hearing Services in Schools, 13,* 144–155.

Katz, J., & Fletcher, C. H. (1982). *Phonemic synthesis: Blending sounds into words.* Vancouver, WA: Precision Acoustics.

The Learning Company. (1993). *Reader Rabbit 2.* Fremont, CA: Author.

Lindamood, C. H., & Lindamood, P. C. (1975). *Auditory discrimination in depth.* Allen, TX: DLM Teaching Resources.

Martin, B., Jr., & Carle, E. (1992). *Brown bear, brown bear, what do you see?* New York: Henry Holt.

Nelson, N. W. (1993). *Childhood language disorders in context: Infancy through adolescence.* New York: Merrill.

Norris, J. (1994). From frog to prince: Using written language as a context for language learning. In K. Butler (Ed.), *Best Practices II: The classroom as an inter-*

vention context (pp. 55–70). Topics in Language Disorders Series. Gaithersburg, MD: Aspen.

Pehrsson, R. S., & Denner, P. R. (1994). Semantic organizers: Implications for reading and writing. In K. Butler (Ed.), *Best Practices II: The classroom as an intervention context* (pp. 71–84). Topics in Language Disorders Series. Gaithersburg, MD: Aspen.

Schuele, C. M. (1994). Emergent literacy: A necessary component of early intervention practices of speech-language pathologists. *Tejas: Texas Journal of Audiology and Speech Pathology, XX,* 2–7.

Swank, L. K., & Catts, H. W. (1994). Phonological awareness and written word decoding. *Language, Speech & Hearing Services in Schools, 25,* 9–14.

9

THE FAST FORWORD PROGRAM

A Clinician's Perspective

THERESA M. CINOTTI
State University of New York at Buffalo

Professionals who work with individuals with language-learning impairments are constantly searching for the cause and the "cure" for these difficulties. One suspected contributing factor to language-learning impairments (LLI) is a central auditory processing disorder (CAPD). A central auditory processing disorder occurs, typically, in the absence of a hearing problem. It is a disruption in the auditory signal as it is processed in the brain. Central auditory processing problems may present with difficulty in perceiving, recalling, or organizing the auditory information received. Without question, difficulties in any of these areas may result in delayed language or learning development. The Buffalo Model of Central Auditory Processing Disorders defines the following four areas of processing difficulties: tolerance-fading memory, decoding, integration, and organization (Katz, Stecker, & Masters, 1994).

A central auditory processing disorder is one probable cause for LLI. The "cure" is more illusive. Language and learning professionals work diligently to provide the most effective therapy, and many programs and theories have proved to be beneficial when working with LLI children. However, the search continues for a therapy tool that will provide rapid and efficacious results. One potential tool is the much anticipated, recently marketed Fast ForWord Program, which targets a variety of receptive language skills, but most apparently, decoding skills. A decoding problem is accompanied by difficulties in discrimination of sounds and a slower processing rate (Katz, Stecker, & Masters, 1994).

Originally named the HAILO program, Scientific Learning Corporation's (SLc) Fast ForWord program was developed through the efforts and research of neuroscientist, Dr. Michael E. Merzenich, cognitive neuroscientist and clinical psychologist; Dr. Paula Tallal; Dr. William Jenkins; and Dr. Steven L. Miller, neuropsychologist. The program is based on the finding that children who have receptive language delays typically process sounds and language at a slower rate than average listeners. This slower processing rate is akin to a central auditory processing disorder in the area of decoding. Using a series of animated computer games, the Fast ForWord program utilizes acoustically altered speech, presented at a slower rate with its most salient acoustic properties amplified. As children learn to discriminate and comprehend speech and language at altered and simplified levels, the computer automatically and incrementally changes the presentation of the stimulus to continually challenge the children. Throughout play, children are constantly rewarded for their success with animations. The goal is that upon completion of the program, children with language-learning impairments will have learned to perceive sounds at a processing rate equal to that of average listeners (Scientific Learning Corporation, February 1997).

Beta studies were conducted with 60 professionals and 500 children. Results of the field trial revealed that over 90 percent of the children achieved improvements in language skills. Children improved an average of 18 months on receptive and expressive language testing after six to eight weeks of training. Some 68 percent of the children were found to move from below-average performance on standardized speech-language testing to performing at the average level and many children moved to the above-average level. (Scientific Learning Corporation, 1997c, 1997d). Follow-up testing was conducted six months following the Beta studies. Results of that testing revealed speech-language gains were maintained. Since the program is relatively new, regression effects have not been studied past six months' postprogram, as of the date of this chapter (Miller & Burns, 1997).

This chapter has been written from the perspective of a speech-language pathologist who has used the Fast ForWord Program with eight children over a two-month period, during the summer of 1997 at a speech-language and hearing clinic. The goal of this chapter is to report on constructs of the program as defined by SLc and to convey one center's experiences during implementation of Fast ForWord in a clinical setting. The data collected on the eight children who participated in this center's administration of the program are minimal, compared to the data col-lected in SLc's expansive Beta studies. However, it is hoped that this chapter will provide insight into the practical applications of the Fast ForWord Program in clinical or educational settings.

THEORY

The Fast ForWord program is based largely on the research of Dr. Paula Tallal, a cognitive neuroscientist and clinical psychologist. Tallal is a professor and co-director of the Center for Molecular and Behavioral Neuroscience and co-director of the Behavior and Neuroscience Doctoral Program at Rutgers University. In addition, she is the executive vice-pres-ident of Scientific Learning Corporation (Scientific Learning Corpora-tion, 1997d).

According to Tallal's research, children with normal intelligence and specific language-learning impairments have a problem in sensory information processing. Specifically, they have trouble processing in 10-millisecond chunks (10 msec = one-hundredth of a second). Speech presented at a normal rate typically allows important information to pass at speeds of 40 msec or less (Scientific Learning Corporation, Febru-ary 1996). Tallal's research supports that children with LLI may be pro-cessing sounds at a much slower rate, often over 200 msec. Therefore, children with language-learning impairments are at a considerable dis-advantage when asked to process information presented at normal rates of speech. This would account for the decreased speech and language comprehension skills usually accompanied by auditory processing diffi-culties. It has been found that as sounds are elongated, the ability for a child with language processing difficulties to accurately perceive that sound increases significantly.

Tallal also accounts for the acoustical alterations that are made to sounds within the context of the Fast ForWord program. She has found that amplification of a sound's most salient features increases how well it can be perceived and allows it to become more distinct from other sim-ilar sounds (Tallal et al., 1996, from Scientific Learning Corporation, Feb-ruary 1997).

Both elongation and amplification of acoustical features has been utilized in the Fast ForWord program to allow for easier discrimination between similar sounds. Children's perception of speech sounds at this altered state can be generalized to normal speech production after a training process that incrementally increases the complexity of the sounds that a child can perceive accurately (Tallal et al., 1996, from Scientific Learning Corporation, February 1997). With increased perception of speech sounds, it is logical to assume that receptive language skills will inherently improve.

Along with Tallal's research on speech perception, Dr. Michael E. Merzenich's research on brain plasticity aided in designing the Fast For-Word Program. Merzenich is a leading expert in brain plasticity, brain mechanisms, and integrative neuroscience. He is a member of the Keck Center for Integrative Neurosciences at the University of California at San Francisco. With over 25 years of experience, Merzenich specializes in the areas of brain science, behavior, and engineering research (Scientific Learning Corporation, 1997).

Research at the University of California at San Francisco (UCSF) revealed that changes in the brain contribute to learning, and these changes can occur throughout one's life time. The life-long capacity for change is called *neuroplasticity* (Scientific Learning Corporation, 1996) Neuroplasticity is an important concept as the Fast ForWord Program focuses on "retraining the brain" to process information. Merzenich developed specific learning routines in his laboratory that were found to be extremely effective in driving brain plasticity for sensory processing (Scientific Learning Corporation, February 1996).

WHO CAN PARTICIPATE

The Fast ForWord program is designed predominantly for children with language-learning impairments, with some flexibility given to clinicians for determining candidacy for programming. Specific suggestions are given for determining if the Fast ForWord Program is appropriate, but professional judgment is highly encouraged for making final decisions regarding candidacy. There are two steps in selecting children for the program. The first step is referring children who would likely benefit. The second step is to complete a thorough speech-language evaluation.

When contemplating whether a child should be referred to the program, it is best to consider who the program was designed for and what children demonstrated the most success with the program during the course of the Beta studies. Generally, the program is designed for children 4 to 12 years of age who present with a language-learning impairment. Among the children who may benefit from Fast ForWord are those who have a receptive or expressive language delay, dyslexia, a language-learning impairment, a sensory integration deficit, a central auditory processing disorder, or a pervasive developmental disorder (Scientific Learning Center, February 1997). It is important to note that children with these types of difficulties participated in Beta study testing, and therefore are included on the list of possible candidates. However, people who have not fit the aforementioned characteristics have very appropriately utilized the Fast ForWord program.

Through various conversations with parents, the Scientific Learning Corporation professional and parent Internet chat room, and Scientific Learning Corporation professional support people, it has been noted that the list of individuals for whom the program benefits is expanding. The program has been utilized with children over age 12, adults, individuals who have learned English as a second language, and individuals with aphasia. Since Scientific Learning Corporation has not collected data on these groups thus far, SLc representatives have cautioned users not to expect the same types of gains as projected by the Beta studies. However, if a client would benefit from improving the processing skills targeted in the program, then Fast ForWord is likely a viable therapy tool. Since the games were designed to entertain children, clinicians are cautioned to consider the maturity level of older clients to ensure that the games are appropriate and stimulating.

Speech-Language Testing

Following referral, an evaluation for programming must be conducted. Very simply, the evaluation criteria states that a child is appropriate for Fast ForWord if he or she scores one standard deviation below the mean on receptive phonology, receptive language, or general language testing. The following tests are suggested by SLc: the Test of Language Comprehension (TLC), the Test of Auditory Comprehension of Language (TACL), the Test of Language Development (TOLD), the Clinical Evaluation of Language Fundamentals (CELF), the Goldman Fristoe Woodcock Test of Auditory Discrimination (GFW), the Preschool Language Scale (PLS), the Token Test for Children, the Test of Auditory Perceptual Skills (TAPS), and the Lindamood Auditory Conceptualization Test (LAC) (Scientific Learning Center, 1997a; February 1997). This list has changed periodically. Some tests have been found more sensitive than others to measure a child's progress on the program. For instance, the TAPS may not be an optimal pretest measure, as it mainly assesses auditory recall skills. Auditory recall tasks are incorporated in the Fast ForWord games, but other areas, such as sound discrimination and sequencing, are more aggressively targeted.

Choosing a general receptive and expressive language measure and a sound discrimination measure is suggested when selecting pretesting material (Miller & Burns, February 1997). As mentioned before, children who perform at least one standard deviation below the mean on a listening comprehension, general language, or receptive phonology test are considered good candidates for the program. Beta studies using the Fast ForWord Program revealed the most drastic speech-language improvements to occur with children who have moderate or severe language delays. Children with mild delays were found to make progress, but because they did not have as far to go, gains were not as dramatic as those of the more significantly language-impaired children. This information is important when deciding programming for those with mild impairments. When counseling parents, it is important to note that although Fast ForWord may be beneficial for children with mild delays, less intensive conventional therapy may be more appropriate for the child's needs.

The STAR

In addition to the standardized testing, SLc requires professionals to administer the Sequential Temporal Analysis Report (STAR). This test is a computer-based test that requires the child to repeat a series of two pitches/sounds. The STAR assesses a child's processing rate and sequencing skills. The test is used for baseline information, as the test itself replicates a processing task that is presented in one of the games the child will play in training.

Subjective Considerations

Although testing is an objective indicator for candidacy, subjective measures or consideration of concomitant factors may be equally beneficial for predicting how appropriate the Fast ForWord Program will be for a particular child. For instance, the Scientific Learning Center (February 1997) notes that a child with attention deficit disorder (ADD), behavior problems, mild mental retardation, contributing medical conditions, or the need for medications may require an extended training time. Subjectively, a clinician may want to consider the maturity level, attention, distractibility, impulsivity, behavior, and physical limitations of a child. For instance, a child whose test scores indicate candidacy for programming may be recommended for more traditional therapy, due to significant impulsivity and behavioral tendencies precluding his or her ability to successfully respond to the games. In many cases, it may be necessary to have a child work in traditional therapy on some of the behaviors that limit their effectiveness with the Fast ForWord games. It may be appropriate to recommend that a child be reevaluated for candidacy following other therapy or intervention. It is crucial to remember that clinical judgment is the most important tool for determining the most beneficial programming for a child.

DESCRIPTION OF PROGRAM

The Design

The Fast ForWord games were designed based on Merzenich's research on brain plasticity and Tallal's research in the area of speech perception and acoustically altered speech (Scientific Learning Center, February 1996). A unique computer algorithm that increases the intensity of the most salient acoustic features of a sound and elongates the brief, rapidly changing components within speech sounds is utilized to enhance a child's perception of speech and language (Scientific Learning Center, February 1996). Using this altered speech, LLI children are given the opportunity to comprehend speech and language at a less challenging level, considering their presumed slower processing rate. Through a series of seven computer games, a child is exposed to stimuli presented to enhance sound discrimination, recall, morphological, semantic, and syntactic skills.

Merzenich's research supporting the use of repetition and reward to change the brain's processing method is taken into account as children are rewarded by a point and token system throughout play. During the games, children are presented with targeted stimuli. As the children demonstrate, through their responses, that they comprehend a stimulus at a particular rate and level of complexity, the computer automatically increases the complexity of the signal.

The Fast ForWord games are programmed to allow the child to maintain an 80 percent success rate with each game. As the child becomes 80 percent proficient in responding to stimuli, the computer increases the difficulty level. If the child is unable to maintain 80 percent success at a particular level, the program automatically adjusts and presents a less challenging stimulus. This method was designed to promote a child's motivation and to allow for optimal opportunity to condition the brain to process various signals at a specific rate of presentation. The Fast ForWord program is different from many other computer programs in that it actually changes with the child. The program adjusts with the performance of the child. It will adapt daily as the child's play advances him or her through the program (Miller & Burns, 1997).

The Games

The Fast ForWord program consists of a series of seven games targeting particular aspects of language processing. The circus sequence game requires the child to reproduce a two-sound sequence by clicking on two buttons that represent the corresponding sounds. Old MacDonald's Flying

Farm requires the child to discriminate between similar phonemes by identifying the moment the successively presented phoneme changes. For the Phoneme Identification Game, the child must identify a targeted phoneme when presented with two similar phonemes. The Phonic Words game requires a child to distinguish between words that differ by only the initial consonant sound. Phonic Match is a game that challenges auditory recall skills as a child is required to match words by selecting a tile that creates a sound, from a grid of 4 to 25 animated tiles. The child must then find the tile that produces the corresponding sound. The Block Commander game utilizes a three-dimensional board filled with circles and squares of various shapes and colors. The child is asked to follow directions, using this board. The Language Comprehension Builder game requires a child to point to a picture from a set of two to four pictures, when presented with various language concepts. Throughout play, children are constantly rewarded for their successes through colorful animations.

During the program, each game lasts 20 minutes. Children who are registered for the Fast ForWord program are asked to comply with a daily game schedule. For optimal advancement of skills, it is suggested that a child play five games a day, one hour and 40 minutes per day, five days per week. The Beta studies indicated that an average of six weeks was necessary for completion of the program. SLc suggests that a child end the program if he or she reaches 90 percent completion in five out of the seven games presented. A child begins play at 0 percent completion for each game. If the child demonstrates comprehension of the information presented, he or she becomes closer to completion daily.

Beta studies and Internet reports from clinicians using Fast ForWord indicate that the program can be completed in as little as four weeks and as much as three months, with more involved children obviously requiring more time to fulfill the stipulations of the program (Miller & Burns, 1997). At times, speech-language improvements can be noted without drastic improvements in the child's program scores. Due to the intensive intervention, speech-language testing may indicate advances, prior to completion of the program, warranting discharge before the five out of the seven games are 90 percent complete. In addition, if the child stagnates at a certain level, termination of the program may be warranted. From discussions with SLc staff and information gained from the SLc chat line, it is encouraged that children be discharged from the program based on professional, clinical judgment.

IMPLEMENTATION

As stated before, the perspective of this chapter is from a speech-language pathologist who has been involved in running the program at a community speech-language and hearing clinic. From that perspective, it can be stated that Fast ForWord requires an extraordinary commitment in time and effort. It is presumed, however, that most professionals will perceive that investment as worthwhile. Fortunately, at this particular center, much support was given administratively and technically. Utilizing a team effort, the center was able to prepare for the great demands of administering this program. As the reader will note, the steps involved in the administration of Fast ForWord are numerous. Since this professional's initial involvement in February 1997, many changes have been made by Scientific Learning Corporation, which will hopefully make initial set-up and administration easier for professionals just starting.

Professional Training

The first step toward administering the program is to attend a Fast For-Word training seminar offered by Scientific Learning Corporation. These seminars are advertised nationally. Seminar information may also be obtained from the Scientific Learning Corporation Website. The current address is http://www.fastforword.com/. After registering, a professional must attend the SLc training seminar, which will provide an overview of the program. Along with the seminar, professionals will receive a training manual that discusses theories and procedures for the Fast ForWord Program. Scientific Learning Corporation sends each professional home from the seminar with a test that must be completed and sent back to SLc. Following successful completion of the test and the signing of a certified professional agreement, SLc registers the professional as a certified provider of the Fast ForWord Program.

Administration Decisions

As a Fast ForWord provider, decisions need to be made about method of administration. Of course, Fast ForWord has a standardized protocol for administration, but there are choices that need to be made regarding the context in which the program is presented. Perhaps the first decision to be made is regarding the number of children that will be working at one time. The games will be played for one hour and 40 minutes a day. If playing in a clinic setting and playing all five of the games successively, it will typically require at least two hours for children to complete their daily play. At the center, which had eight children in the summer of 1997, two hours a day were allotted per Fast ForWord session so that children could take a snack break between the third and fourth games. This time will certainly vary, depending on the needs of the children.

Physical Accommodations

After deciding the number of children that will play at one time, the physical layout of the facility should be considered. Several children can play the games at one time in one room, depending on the set-up of the room and the behaviors of the children playing. All children must wear headphones to play, therefore their games should not interfere with the play of the other children. If using one room for several children, it is recommended that visual barriers be placed between the children to reduce their tendency to look around and be distracted by others' play. In some cases, separate rooms are more feasible, since some children may have a tendency to distract others.

With the eight children at the speech-language and hearing center, it was found that when children required additional instruction from the speech-language pathologist, the interaction at times interfered with the play of other children. For children with significant needs, playing in a separate room may be considered. A group play area may be more motivating for children who can play the games relatively independently with minimal verbal interaction with the clinician. It was found at the center that the children valued the peer interaction and enjoyed talking about the games with their new friends.

Monitoring Decisions

Another decision to be made is to determine who will be monitoring the actual playing of the games. SLc requires a certified professional to supervise each child's progress through the games, but it allows monitors to watch the actual daily play. The trained and certified professional is responsible for training a monitor to guide the children through their daily game routines. Monitors are also responsible for encouraging the children and providing positive reinforcement. Although the games are designed to be played independently, a monitor is necessary to ensure compliance with the games, especially if a group of children are playing at one time.

The Room

After decisions are made regarding the number of children to play, group versus individual play, and monitoring, room considerations can be made. Of course, the size of the room will depend on the number of children playing. Group rooms should have visual barriers to deter from distractions when playing. There needs to be ample room for a monitor to move around the room unobtrusively. Perhaps, most importantly, the room must be Internet ready. If there are multiple computers in one room, a network connection would probably be most beneficial.

Computers

The final and most crucial preparation to be made is selection, purchase (if necessary), and set-up of the computers. This may be easier said than done, depending on the computer resources available at a particular site. The Fast ForWord games run off CD-ROM technology and require the use of the Internet to analyze performance. Therefore, a powerful computer is necessary to run the program. Recently, SLc has made the program available for both Macintosh and PC systems. Prior to July 1997, the program was only available for Macintosh computers. Given this change, computer acquisition may be easier for professionals. However, there are still specifications that must be met for the Fast ForWord Program to be run on a computer. Although requirements may change as the Fast ForWord Program continues to develop, the following computer specifications (Scientific Learning Corporation, 1997b) are necessary as of the date of this chapter:

Windows 95

Computer:	PC-compatible
Processor:	Pentium
Memory:	16 MB
Operating System:	Windows 95
Sound:	16-bit sound card
CD-ROM:	Quad-speed (4x) CD-ROM drive
Modem:	28.8 modem or faster
Connectivity:	Internet connection from an Internet Service Provider (ISP)
Web Browser:	Netscape Navigator 3.01 or higher, or Microsoft Internet Explorer 3.02 or higher
Headphones:	Closed-type stereo headphones

Mac OS

Computer:	Apple Macintosh or Macintosh Compatible
Processor:	Power PC 601, 603, or 604 processor
Memory:	16 MB
Operating System:	Mac OS 7.5.5 or higher
Sound:	16-bit sound (audio in and out)
CD-ROM:	Quad-speed (4x) CD-ROM drive
Connectivity:	Internet connection from an Internet Service Provider (ISP)
Web Browser:	Netscape Navigator 3.01 or higher, or Microsoft Internet Explorer 3.01 or higher
Headphones:	Closed-type stereo headphones

Meeting the computer requirements may be the most costly part of a clinician or agency's investment. Some facilities may be computer ready, making start-up of the Fast ForWord Program more feasible. For those starting from scratch, the purchase and preparation of the computers may be the most time-consuming precursor to administering the program. If certified professionals are not familiar with various computer operations or Internet functions, it may be beneficial to hire a computer consultant to aid in the technological set-up of the program. At the center described here, computer experts were already on staff to attend to technical needs. Even with this support, this unique program required a great deal of time and effort to set up for most effective operation. Technological support is provided through SLc to aid those setting up the program. After the computer technology is in place, it would behoove professionals and monitors to practice the games and various maneuvers that they will have to complete regularly when actually administering the program to children.

As the reader may have surmised thus far, the Fast ForWord program requires a substantial commitment by the professional. Set-up for the program requires a significant investment in time, energy, and money. This commitment must continue when the program is actually implemented with children.

General Implementation

After the facility and equipment are prepared for the program, testing of children may begin. The clinician should use the specified criteria and clinical judgment to determine a child's candidacy for the program. The child must be registered with SLc on the Internet so that they may take the STAR test. Following testing, STAR performance must be uploaded to SLc and then downloaded back to the professional with SLc's interpretation of the STAR results.

Once parents and professionals decide that a child will participate in the program, the child must be registered as an active client with SLc. In addition, the parents must sign a contract with SLc as well as pay a program fee directly to SLc. The program fee is currently $850.00, payable directly to SLc for an individual's right to utilize the program and receive SLc's data analysis services. This cost is separate from the additional fee charged by the professional administering the program.

Only the child registered may play the games, since the program becomes automatically customized during play, according to the needs of the child. Once the child is registered and activated by SLc, he or she may begin play on the games. For the first three days of play, the child will begin playing just three games. On the fourth and fifth days, four games will be played. From then on, the child will be required to play five games per day, 20 minutes per game, five days per week. This game schedule is highly encouraged by SLc. Compliance to this schedule will increase the chance of advancement using Fast ForWord. Since the program requires at least 140 minutes of play per day, the child may quit between games, allowing for a break, and then complete games at a later time. Once a game is started, it cannot be stopped until 15 minutes have elapsed. There are seven games in the program. Generally, a child must reach 90 percent completion in five out of the seven games to reach discharge criteria. Scientific Learning Corporation notes that children typically reach this criteria six to eight weeks following initiation of the program. This time will vary according to the functional level of each child.

On a daily basis, monitors should encourage the children to attend to the program and should provide positive reinforcement. As children complete their games, their information is uploaded via the Internet to SLc. Information can then be downloaded from SLc in the form of text and graphs. A child's progress on each game can be seen daily. Certified professionals are responsible for reading the data and interpreting the information. The responsible professional will give recommendations regarding additional needs of the child and will counsel the parent regarding progress and projected discharge. The professional will also monitor speech-language gains.

Special Adaptations

The previously mentioned procedures are those that professionals may implement with the majority of the children. For children who present with more clinical challenges, adaptations may need to be made. For instance, in the work at this professional's center, it was found that some children needed a clinician or monitor sitting next to them to remind them to continue or to help them with strategies to enhance game play. Monitors reminded children to reauditorize or use rehearsal techniques when completing the following-directions tasks, language comprehension tasks, or sequencing tasks for the block commander, language comprehension builder, and circus sequence games, respectively. It was noted, for one child, that impulsivity appeared to be a problem when responding to the circus sequence game. It was necessary for this child to point to the responses on the screen rather than use the mouse, since his impulsivity increased with the fast clicking of the mouse.

It was also necessary to provide picture cues for two children who had difficulty understanding the concept of high sounds versus low sounds. One child chose an elephant to represent high tones because of the high-pitched trumpet sound it produces. He chose an owl to represent low tones due to its low-pitched "hoo" sound. These pictures were taped onto the computer screen to help the child define a relationship between the sounds he was perceiving. In addition, tactile cues were given to assist in defining the concepts of high and low. Using a chat room conversation suggestion, a feather was used to help the child relate to higher sounds and rough sand paper was used to help the child relate to low sounds. Additional training was also provided to enhance one child's pitch perception. His parents worked at home and in our center with a musical keyboard, playing pitch-sequencing games.

We also found that simple adaptations, such as providing more comfortable seating, enhanced children's attention to the games. In a group room, it was helpful to have a splicer on the headphone jack so the monitor or clinician could plug into a child's computer and listen to the stimuli to which the child was responding correctly or incorrectly. With this knowledge, the monitor is able to provide feedback immediately to the child so he or she can become aware of play strategies. For example, when playing the phonic match game, which requires a child to click on a square from a selection of 4 to 25 squares, hear an acoustically altered word, and find the square that produces the matching word, the clinician can help the child to systematically sample words rather than using a random guessing technique. Although these techniques are not specifically suggested in Fast ForWord literature, it is the responsibility of the professional to provide the child with the greatest opportunity to attend to and respond to the stimuli presented.

SLc also allows for the Fast ForWord Program to be administered at home. In these cases, parents must be trained to monitor the child's play. Speech-language pathologists are required to review information, monitor progress, make suggestions, consult with parents, and assist with programming decisions. Although this home therapy is often more convenient, SLc reports the best results with on-site programming, predominantly due to compliance and motivational issues (Miller & Burns, 1997).

RESULTS

As mentioned before, this clinician's experience with working on the Fast ForWord program with eight children is minimal, compared to the hundreds of children who participated in the program during the Beta studies. Therefore, the information that follows regarding the results of these eight children should be guardedly interpreted, as it represents one center's experience with a small number of children.

Performance on the Program

The first measure of performance to discuss is the actual completion criteria. As previously noted, discharge is suggested when a child reaches 90 percent completion in five out of the seven games played. Beta studies revealed completion to occur, on average, four to six weeks after initiation of the program. SLc suggests to expect six to eight weeks for completion of the program during clinical application. The information that is available on the children at this clinician's center reflects performance after eight weeks of play.

After six weeks of play, only one child had reached the suggested completion criteria. She actually reached completion after four weeks of play, but demonstrated that she still had room for growth in the remaining areas. She was discharged after a total of six weeks of play, achieving over 90 percent completion in six of the seven games. On the one game that she did not attain completion, she had achieved 90 percent completion at one point, but did not maintain her score for more than one day.

After seven weeks of play, another child was near completion. He had reached at least 90 percent completion on four of the seven games and was at 89 percent completion for a fifth game. After eight weeks, this child was ready for discharge.

Following eight weeks of play, a third child reached 90 percent completion on four of the seven games. Continued play was recommended.

Of the five remaining children, 90 percent completion was achieved in three of seven games for one child, two of seven games for another child, one of seven games for two of the children, and zero out of the seven games for the last child after eight weeks. For all of these children, continued play on the Fast ForWord program was recommended.

Speech-Language Results

Only three of the eight children worked with achieved the completion criteria within the eight-week period that was suggested to be expected, but preliminary speech-language testing indicated that children made significant gains despite the fact that they did not reach SLc's suggested completion criteria.

Of the two children who reached completion criteria, significant speech-language gains were documented with follow-up testing. The first child who was discharged after six weeks improved from displaying a mild to moderate receptive language delay and a severe expressive language delay on the Clinical Evaluation of Language Fundamentals–3rd edition (CELF-3) to demonstrating a mild receptive and expressive language delay. Her age-equivalent score increased from 5 years, 0 months to 6 years, 0 months, indicating a 12-month gain in language skills as measured by the CELF-3. On the Lindamood Test of Auditory Conceptualization (LAC), this child improved from scoring at the first half of the year at the kindergarten level to performing at the second half of the year at the first-grade level, one point away from scoring at a second-grade level.

The second child who completed the program after eight weeks of play also demonstrated significant language gains. This child—who originally displayed severe delays in comprehension of concepts and directions and word classes, a moderate delay in comprehension of semantic relationships, and a severe delay in sentence recall ability—improved to exhibit moderate delays in comprehension of concepts and directions and word classes, a mild delay in sentence recall skills, and age-appropriate comprehension of semantic relationships. Further services were recommended to address remaining needs in conventional therapy.

Some of the children who had not yet completed the program by the eight-week point were tested at six and seven weeks of play. Gains were demonstrated on that testing, even though they had not completed the training program. The child who did not reach completion criteria on any of the games increased his receptive language score from exhibiting an overall severe delay on the Test of Auditory Comprehension of Language–Revised (TACL-R) to displaying overall low-average but age-appropriate receptive language skills.

The child who reached completion criteria on one game initially displayed an overall severe receptive language delay on the CELF-3. After seven weeks, he demonstrated borderline age-appropriate comprehension on the CELF-3. On the sentence structure subtest, he improved from scoring in the moderate delay range to scoring in the above-average range. On the concepts and directions subtest, he improved from exhibiting a severe delay to showing a moderate delay. On the word classes subtest, he improved from scoring in the severe range of delay to scoring in the mild range of delay. The child who reached 90 percent completion on three games improved from displaying moderate delays on all three subtests of the CELF-3 to exhibiting a moderate delay on the concept and directions subtest and age-appropriate skills on the word classes and semantic relationships subtests, after seven weeks of play.

Posttesting data were not available on the other children in the program at the time this chapter was written. Of the children posttested, all made language gains, some more significant than others. Even those who did not complete the Fast ForWord program were found to benefit by their exposure to the games.

Parent Impression

Parents have been another source of information regarding the success of the program. Of the eight children, six had parents who reported noticeable changes at home. One had noted minimal changes and one was unsure if any changes in language occurred. The following are quotes from parents regarding the changes noted: "She is saying something new everyday"; "He is able to follow directions"; "He still has trouble following the whole direction, but he is getting more right"; "He sounds like he is speaking more clearly"; "She is answering the telephone and she never wanted to talk on the phone before"; "After not seeing my son for a month, I can really tell that this has made a difference."

Correlation between SLc Study and Speech-Language Clinic Results

Overall, speech-language gains noted in the small clinical therapy group seem to correlate well with the expected gains that SLc notes in its literature. The children at this clinician's speech-language and hearing clinic performed differently than the average child in the Beta study with respect to the length of time required to reach suggested completion criteria. Beta study participants averaged six weeks to complete the program. The majority of the clinic's children required over eight weeks to complete the program.

General Impressions

Overall, this clinician is satisfied with the results of the Fast ForWord program. This program targets many of the receptive phonology, receptive language, syntactic, and semantic skills that a speech-language pathologist would target in conventional therapy. The theories behind the design and implementation of the Fast ForWord program highly correlate with accepted and effective methods utilized in traditional therapy. This program appears to be more effective, in some very specific areas, for rapid gains due its advantage of being able to instantaneously track the child's progress, adapt during play, and consistently reward for success. In addition, the program is naturally stimulating to a child because of its method of presentation.

The Fast ForWord program can be viewed as a very effective tool for enhancing decoding skills and various receptive language skills of LLI children. It appears to be a capable way of training some basic underlying receptive phonological skills that can be used as building blocks to acquire enhanced receptive and expressive language skills. It is hoped that the cost to both parents and professionals will be lessened in the future so that Fast ForWord can be more feasibly and equitably administered to those who demonstrate a need.

Although this program appears to be highly effective for many children, it should not be considered a cure-all for language delays. Fast ForWord targets discrete skills presented in a structured setting. It is likely that after completion of the Fast ForWord program, the child will require follow-up speech-language services to work on skills necessary for functional comprehension and expression in home and school settings. It is reasonable to assume that additional receptive or expressive language, pragmatic, or speech improvement therapy may be necessary during or after the Fast ForWord Program. Hopefully, with the improvements in processing made during the course of the Fast ForWord Program, further speech-language acquisition will be made easier when conventional speech-language therapy is resumed. It is also important to note that the program is not for every child. Clinical judgment for selection of Fast ForWord participants is crucial.

SUMMARY

Scientific Learning Corporation's Fast ForWord Program is a unique computer-based receptive language intervention tool designed from the research of Dr. Paula Tallal and Dr. Michael Merzenich. Although the program targets a variety of language skills, it devotes much energy to enhancing discrimination and processing rates, typically associated with decoding disorders. Fast ForWord was originally developed for enhancing the skills of LLI children; however, since its clinical use, other groups have been found to benefit from Fast ForWord intervention. Beta studies conducted with 500 children between 4 and 12 years of age revealed that over 90 percent of the children achieved improvements in language skills. Children improved an average of 18 months on receptive and expressive language testing after six to eight weeks of training consisting of 1 hour and 40 minutes of play per day, 5 days per week (Scientific Learning Corporation, 1997).

Use of the Fast ForWord Program with eight children at a community speech-language and hearing clinic revealed language gains for the participants. However, the time involved proved to be greater than eight weeks for the majority of the children. Although this program seems to be efficacious for many LLI children, its use should be carefully considered with each child. Scientific Learning Corporation's candidate criteria should be taken into account as well as professional and clinical judgment when determining the most appropriate programming.

The Fast ForWord Program is highly successful in improving targeted receptive language skills, and its use can potentially enhance further language growth, following completion of the program. Fast ForWord should by no means be considered the "cure" for LLI; however, it can be viewed as a good start for many of the children who fit the qualifications for candidacy. As its design facilitates the development of decoding skills, it can, in all likelihood, do what its creators claim. It may very well retrain the brain to process information, thereby decreasing the burden and disadvantage possessed by many LLI children.

As the administration and use of the Fast ForWord Program becomes more financially feasible to professionals and parents, professionals may be able to more readily incorporate the program into their therapeutic repertoire for use prior to, in conjunction with, or after conventional methods. It is hoped that research continues to support this program's efficacy with children in clinical and educational settings.

REFERENCES

Katz, J., Stecker, N., & Masters, M. G. (1994, March). *Central auditory processing: A coherent approach.* American Speech-Language-Hearing Association Presentation, Albuquerque, NM.

Miller, S., & Burns, M. (1997, February). Scientific Learning Corporation: Training Seminar.

Scientific Learning Corporation. (1996, February). Website: The Scientific Basis of HAILO.

Scientific Learning Corporation. (1997, February). Training Seminar Manual.

Scientific Learning Corporation. (1997a). Procedural Manual for Professionals.

Scientific Learning Corporation. (1997b). Technical Manual for Parents.

Scientific Learning Corporation. (1997c). Website: "Management."

Scientific Learning Corporation. (1997d). Website: "Frequently Asked Questions."

Tallal, P., Miller, S., Jenkins, B., & Merzenich, M. (1997). *The role of temporal processing in developmental language-based learning disorder: Research and clinical implications.* Scientific Learning Corporation, Training Seminar Manual.

10

IS AUDITORY INTEGRATION TRAINING AN EFFECTIVE TREATMENT FOR CHILDREN WITH CENTRAL AUDITORY PROCESSING DISORDERS?

KAREN A. YENCER
State University of New York at Buffalo

Central auditory processing disorder (CAPD), the inability to efficiently perceive or process sound, including speech, has been linked with learning disabilities (Katz & Illmer, 1972; Pinheiro, 1977; Johnson et al., 1981; Musiek et al., 1982; Jerger et al., 1987), deficits in reading accuracy and reading comprehension (Mulder & Curtin, 1955; Flynn & Byrne, 1970; Katz & Wilde, 1985), poor spelling ability (Bannatyne & Wichiarajote, 1969; Witkin, 1971), and expressive and receptive language difficulties (Sloan, 1980; Butler, 1983; Young, 1983; Howard & Hulit, 1992). In recent years, a great deal of progress has been made in identifying various areas of CAPD and associated academic deficiencies. There also has been considerable interest in management or remediation strategies for CAPD (Willeford & Burleigh, 1985; Jirsa, 1992; Schneider, 1992; Katz & Cohen, 1985). To date, many of the therapy procedures do not have empirical support to show their effectiveness.

TRADITIONAL METHODS TO REMEDIATE CAPD

Traditional therapies for CAPD have typically been administered over periods of months or even years. Phonemic synthesis therapy, a treatment for an area of CAPD deficit characterized by inability to efficiently recognize and use phonemes, has met with some success (Katz & Burge, 1971; Katz & Medol, 1972; Katz, 1983). Similarly, a recently developed training program that alters the timing and intensity of speech components appears to hold promise for children who are not able to follow rapidly changing phonetic elements of speech (Merzenich et al., 1996; Tallal et al., 1996). Although therapy methods exist for treating other areas of CAPD—for example, speech-in-noise desensitization training and auditory memory exercises or therapy that focuses on following oral directions—empirical studies have not determined the efficacy of such methods.

The purpose of this chapter is to explain why the central auditory system would likely change following a training program, explain how change may be measured, and describe an empirical study of auditory integration training (AIT), a therapy method that has been reported to be of benefit to individuals with CAPD.

WHY ARE POSITIVE EFFECTS FROM THERAPY PLAUSIBLE?

Neural Plasticity

Past and present research indicates that not only is sound stimulation necessary to the development of auditory function but it can also change both anatomy and physiology of the central nervous system (CNS). In animal models, evidence of neural plasticity, the capability of the CNS to change or be modified (Milgram et al., 1987), has been reported at several levels of the auditory brain stem (Webster, 1983; Webster & Webster, 1977, 1978, 1979; Evans et al., 1983) and in the auditory cortex (Robertson & Irvine, 1989). A subtype of neural plasticity, developmental neural plasticity, is described as modification that is largely mediated by internal events such as chemical medium and growth patterns of surrounding cells (Milgram et al., 1987). Studies of the somatosensory system in humans suggest that developmental neural plasticity exists in infancy and late childhood (Woods & Teuber, 1978), when dendrites and synaptic connections continue to grow and form (Huttenlocher, 1990).

In addition to developmental neural plasticity, CNS modification occurs in response to general levels of environmental stimulation, called experience-dependent plasticity (Milgram et al., 1987). In animal models, changes in neural growth (Rosensweig, 1984) and the size and number of synapses in the CNS are reported in response to general levels of environmental stimulation (Milgram et al., 1987). In addition, human studies support the idea that external stimulation is necessary for the growth and development of the auditory nervous system (Ryals et al., 1991).

Benefits of Stimulation to the Auditory System

From another perspective, it has been shown in animal models that auditory stimulation by means of moderate-level sound exposures, that do not result in permanent changes in hearing thresholds, may be beneficial. "Conditioning" noise exposures have been shown to have a protective effect from future noise exposures (Canlon et al., 1988; Campo et al., 1991), increase the function of outer hair cells (OHCS) (Canlon et al., 1992), and may narrow evoked potential tuning curves (Nast, 1992), implying improved frequency selectivity and discrimination. Based on the evidence, it is plausible that a therapy method that provides considerable auditory stimulation could benefit auditory system function in humans, especially during childhood, when neural plasticity is likely to be greatest.

METHODS TO ASSESS THE EFFICACY OF CAPD THERAPY

Behavioral Assessment

Central auditory processing ability is typically assessed using a test battery that evaluates several areas or subskills of CAPD (Ferre & Wilber, 1986; Ivey & Willeford, 1988; Katz, 1992; Baran & Musiek, 1994). For example, administration of the Staggered Spondaic Word (SSW)—a test that assesses the individual's ability to process competing words—in addition to filtered or time-altered speech tests, a speech-in-noise test, a pitch sequencing test, and tests that challenge the listener's ability to recognize and manipulate speech sounds, are common approaches to CAPD assessment.

Electrophysiological Assessment

Electrophysiological tests assess the timing and magnitude of neural responses, typically to nonspeech auditory stimuli, and have been shown to be sensitive to changes in neural function that correlate with changes in auditory processing. In contrast to behavioral tests, physiological measurements could reveal subtle changes in neural function associated with CAPD that might not be reflected in behavioral responses. Therefore, a combination of physiological and behavioral methods would yield a more complete picture, potentially relating the two perspectives.

Recently, recording of the auditory brain stem response (ABR) and the P300 (P3) event-related potential have been used for clinical and research purposes to measure the function of auditory neural pathways and processes from the brain stem to the auditory cortex. Electrophysiological measurement has been shown to be useful in differentiating children with normal hearing who have a history of otitis media with effusion (OME) from children without histories of OME. Folsom, Weber, and Thompson (1983) found significantly longer ABR wave III and V absolute latencies and wave I-III and III-V interwave latencies in children who had experienced at least six episodes of otitis media with effusion. Children with histories of OME have been shown to have decreased auditory processing skills, including poor performance on low-pass filtered speech (Ferre & Wilber, 1986), dichotic listening, competing message tasks (Jerger et al., 1983), binaural fusion tests (Brandes & Ehinger, 1981; Welsh et al., 1983), and phonological development tasks (Paden et al., 1987, 1989; Roberts et al., 1988).

Children with confirmed CAPD have also been differentiated from children who had no CAPD using electrophysiological tests (Jirsa & Clontz, 1990; Ivey, 1992; Jirsa, 1992). Jirsa and Clontz (1990) demonstrated that children identified with CAPD had smaller amplitude and longer latency P3 event-related potentials compared to non-CAPD controls. In a second study, Jirsa (1992) showed that, following clinical intervention, P3 amplitude increased, latency decreased, and scores improved compared to a CAPD control group that did not receive intervention. Therefore, P3 appears to be a suitable evoked potential to assess to monitor changes in auditory processing ability.

AUDITORY INTEGRATION TRAINING (AIT)

Auditory integration training (AIT), developed by Berard (1993), presents the recipient with 10 hours of loud, frequency-altered music over a 10-day period. The user's guide for one of several available devices used to administer AIT states that "frequencies are varied over a 40 dB range at a random rate" (BGC Enterprises, 1993, p. 8) by the device. The learning-disabled population is the primary population treated by Berard with AIT (Berard, 1993). Berard states that the AIT method is effective in remediating hearing "distortions." These are associated with deficits in discrimination and recognition of speech sounds, distractability from noise, ability to follow spoken language, and delays or unusually rapid responses to speech or environmental sounds. These deficits, reportedly remediated by AIT, are also characteristics of individuals with CAPD.

Berard theorizes that AIT is effective because of the added "work" the cochlea must do to listen to the loud, frequency-altered music. He believes that AIT forces the auditory system to respond to a greater than normal frequency and intensity range of sound, ultimately enabling the listener to perceive all frequencies equally well (Berard, 1993).

Berard's theory and the AIT method have met with a considerable amount of skepticism from the scientific community. To date, there are no empirical studies providing objective evidence of the effectiveness of AIT to remediate auditory processing deficits. However, several recently published studies suggest that AIT may be associated with positive changes in speech-language, hearing, and behavior in individuals with autism (Rimland & Edelson, 1994; Monville & Nelson, 1994). In addition, many positive anecdotal reports and a number of unpublished clinical studies suggest that AIT may be a beneficial treatment for attention deficits and CAPD as well as autism. There is presently a great interest in determining, by empricial methods, if AIT is a beneficial treatment and, if so, for what specific problem areas or populations. The American Speech-Language-Hearing Association (ASHA) (1994) has called for well-controlled study of the effectiveness of AIT for specific populations, including those with learning disorders.

This study looked at behavioral and electrophysiological test data from children before and after a standard 10-day course of AIT in order to determine if this treatment improved deficient CAPD skills, or resulted in changes in neural function that may be associated with deficient auditory processing. Three groups were evaluated: (1) an experimental group that received AIT, (2) a placebo group that received regular music, and (3) a nontreatment control group.

Method

Subjects

There were 36 children, ages 7 to 9 years (10 females, distributed among groups) who participated in this study. The children were selected based on scores that were significantly below average on the SSW test and one or both of the Phonemic Synthesis test and a speech-in-noise test. Based on this selection criterion and the listening and learning difficulties described by parents, the subjects represented a group of children with significant CAP difficulties. Children with autism, pervasive developmental disorder (PDD), multiple handicaps, or other known neurological or developmental disabilities were excluded. Children with known attention deficits were not excluded because these problems are commonly associated with CAPD (Keller, 1992; Tillery, 1992). To exclude them would have eliminated a significant percentage of subjects and skewed the sample. Furthermore, the design of the study diminished detrimental effects of attention problems as each child served as his or her own baseline. Eight of the children (distributed among groups) had known attention deficits. One child in the placebo group took methylphenidate for attention deficit disorder (ADD) throughout his participation in the study, including during the test sessions.

Puretone thresholds of 20 dB HL or better were required at 500, 1,000, 2,000 and 4,000 Hz for participation to assure that hearing was normal and to set presentation levels for the behavioral CAP tests. Tympanometric results were used to determine an absence of active middle ear pathology that might affect the children's performance. Normal middle ear function, peak middle ear pressure of no less than −150 daPa, and static acoustic admittance of no less than .2 mmho were required (ASHA, 1989) with the following exception. Four subjects with unilateral or bilateral patent tympanostomy tubes were included in the control group because this group received no treatment. For these four subjects, tympanostomy tube patency was verified by Type B (flat) tympanograms and physical ear canal volumes greater than 2.5 cm^3.

Behavioral Tests of Auditory Processing

The behavioral tests used to assess the children's auditory processing of speech included a dichotic listening task, a phonemic decoding and sound blending task, and a speech-in-noise discrimination task. The SSW and the Phonemic Synthesis tests were administered following standard procedures (Katz, 1987; Katz & Harmon, 1982). A speech-in-noise discrimination test was administered using monsyllabic words and speech-spectrum noise presented at a +10 dB signal-to-noise ratio. These tests were selected because there have been various claims that AIT improves the ability to process spoken language and to decode or discriminate speech sounds, and is associated with decreased distraction when listening in the presence of background noise.

Electrophysiological Tests

The advantage of electrophysiological tests is that practice, learning, or placebo effects are not of concern and are controlled by the nature of these tests. The brain potentials evaluated in this study were the auditory brain stem response (ABR) and the P300 (P3) event-related potential.

Auditory Brain Stem Response (ABR). For the ipsilateral auditory brain stem responses (ABR), the mid-forehead (Fpz) served as the active site (noninverting electrode). Ipsilateral mastoids and the inion served as the inverting and common electrode sites, respectively. Stimuli were rarefaction clicks of 100 microsecond duration presented individually to each ear at 80dB nHL at a rate of 11.1/second. This presentation rate is essentially the same as rates previously used by Lenhardt (1981) and Kraus and colleagues (1993), who noted delayed ABRs in individuals with CAPDs. From 100 to 3,000 Hz analog bandpass filters were employed. Two trials of 2,000 artifact-free samples were collected for each ear.

P300 (P3). The same P3 recording parameters used by Jirsa and Clontz (1990) to demonstrate prolonged latencies and decreased amplitudes for children with CAPD compared to children without CAP disorders were employed with two exceptions. Jirsa and Clontz used a binaural presentation and a 1 Hz to 100 Hz filter bandpass. In this study, single channel, contralateral, P3 recordings were obtained from vertex (noninverting), mastoid (inverting), and mid-forehead (common) electrode sites. The filter bandpass was set at 1 Hz to 30 Hz because the P3 response is primarily in the frequency region below 30 Hz (Sayers et al., 1974).

Computer-controlled random presentation of 2,000 Hz tone-bursts (infrequent tones) embedded in a steady train of 1,000 Hz tone-bursts (frequent tones) were used to elicit the P3 responses. The frequent and infrequent stimulus responses were averaged separately. Two trials of approximately 100 artifact-free samples were obtained for each ear. The children's attention to the P3 task was maintained by having them count the infrequent stimuli in their head while also using a manual counter. Accuracy was less than 10 percent error for all data included in the analysis.

Fisher's Auditory Problems Checklist (FAPC)
The 25 items that comprise Fisher's Auditory Problems Checklist (FAPC) (Fisher, 1980) describe listening/learning behaviors related to auditory processing. One parent of each subject was asked to respond to the FAPC by checking behaviors observed in their child over the previous week. Based on parents' responses to the FAPC, Rimland and Edelson (1994) reported a positive trend in reduction of these listening/learning problem behaviors following AIT for individuals with autism.

The Standard Progressive Matrices Test
The Standard Progressive Matrices Test (Raven, 1990) was administered to determine if a Hawthorne effect might account for perceived benefits

from AIT—that is, improvement due to reasons other than experimental treatment (e.g., subject/parent expectations, more confidence, more attention, etc.). This visual reasoning test, consisting of a set of designs for which a missing insert must be chosen, is considered a measure of intelligence. Successful performance on the Standard Progressive Matrices does not depend on proficient auditory or speech-language skills (Raven et al., 1985). Therefore, a significant degree of improvement was not expected following AIT.

Procedure

Subjects were assigned to the experimental (E), placebo (P), or control (C) group after being matched by age and SSW total number of errors. This ensured that there were no statistically significant differences between the groups on these two variables. The groups were also compared with respect to the remaining behavioral or electrophysiological variables. No significant differences were found between groups. Experimental and placebo subjects (and their parents) were not informed as to which group they had been assigned.

Because of the number of tests administered, subjects were tested in two 90-minute sessions. After the initial testing, the experimental and placebo groups listened to 10 hours of the modified (AIT) or regular (passed through the AIT device without modification) music, respectively. Two 30-minute sessions a day were required over a 10-day period. The control group did not receive any special treatment. Subjects were retested seven weeks after the initial test session (approximately four weeks after receiving AIT). A decrease in problem behaviors following AIT was reported by Rimland and Edelson (1994) based on parents' responses to the FAPC at this time period. The study paradigm is shown in Figure 10.1.

Experimenter bias was controlled by having two judges coscore 100 percent of the CAP behavioral tests. The second judge was blind to subject condition. ABR latencies for all traces included in the study were marked by one judge. A second judge, blind to subject condition, marked latencies for 20 percent of the traces, randomly selected from the initial and follow-up test sessions for each of the three groups. Statistical analysis of the ABR latencies chosen by the two judges revealed no difference (matched pairs t-test, .05 level of confidence). Therefore, the latencies determined by the first judge were deemed accurate and used in the ABR data analysis. For the P3 response, P3 was defined as the maxima in the 250 to 588 msec time window from stimulus onset. This method of identification, termed "P3 Max" (Polich, 1993) obviated the need for coscorers.

FIGURE 10.1   Study Paradigm

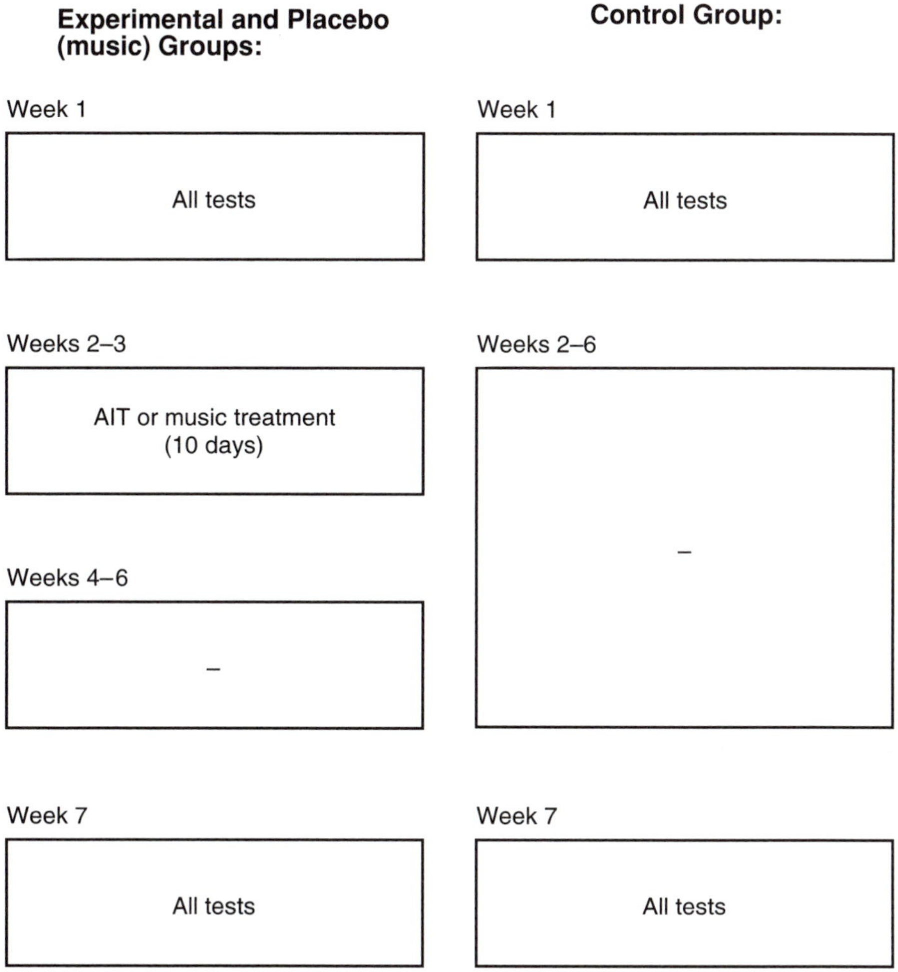

Experimental and Placebo (music) Groups:

Week 1

| All tests |

Weeks 2–3

| AIT or music treatment (10 days) |

Weeks 4–6

| – |

Week 7

| All tests |

Control Group:

Week 1

| All tests |

Weeks 2–6

| – |

Week 7

| All tests |

Auditory Integration Training (AIT).   The BGC Audio Effects Generator Model AT102-1 (BGC Enterprises, Inc.) and Koss HV/PRO headphones, provided with the device, were used to modify compact disc music for the experimental group and to present the nonaltered music to the placebo group. The experimental group received the AIT treatment following the Berard Method (S. Edelson, personal communication, February 28, 1994), with the exception that the device's notch filters were not activated because Rimland and Edelson (1994) found that use of filters during AIT did not result in a difference in treatment outcome. A second exception to the Berard method was that children were allowed to engage in quiet activities such as drawing, building with blocks, or playing with dolls.

The BGC device settings were maintained at "modulate high" and "modulate low," simultaneously, over the 10 hours of therapy for the experimental group. The average sound pressure level of the BGC device output through the HV/PRO headphones over a 10-hour period was measured. Based on this measurement, the experimental subjects received the AIT music at an approximate average sound pressure level (SPL) of 81.2 dB(A), with peak intensity of 110.5 dB(A), an intensity level that was loud as recommended by the Berard method (S. Edelson, personal communication, February 28, 1992). The placebo group was presented with the nonaltered music at an average sound pressure level of 80.4 dB(A), with peak intensity of 110.5 dB(A), determined by similar measurement of the nonmodified music. These sound pressure levels were well below levels that would likely affect the children's hearing.

Analysis and Results

Subjects' initial test results were compared to posttreatment test results (second test results for the control group). For all tests, statistical comparisons were made between groups E and P and between groups E and C. Based on paired t-tests and a .01 level of confidence, no statistically significant differences were found between groups for any of the behavioral tests or subtest conditions or for the electrophysiological test results. The .01 level of confidence was chosen over the .05 level of confidence in order to avoid identifying a significant difference, in error, when none existed. This could occur when using the less strict .05 level of confidence to compute a large number of t-tests within a study.

Behavioral Auditory Processing Tests

For the SSW test, consistent, nonstatistically significant decreases in number of errors for individual conditions were found for each of the three groups. That is, scores improved by similar degrees for each of the groups for the RC and LC conditions as well as total number of SSW errors. The total number of errors decreased by about 3.5 for group E and C and by about 7 errors for group P at the time of posttest (week 7), as shown in Table 10.1.

The general improvement in SSW total number of errors and subcondition errors is a revealing finding. Improvement was reported in SSW scores, speech-in-noise scores, and scores for other behavioral CAP tests

TABLE 10.1   Means and Standard Deviations[1] for the Behavioral Test Results

Group	Experimental	Placebo	Control
SSW Total Number of Errors:			
Pre	27.00 (15.3)	28.17 (16.8)	25.92 (13.2)
Post	23.5 (18.4)	21.25 (14.2)	22.25 (15.8)
Phonemic Synthesis Number Correct:			
Pre	15.9 (6.8)	16.7 (5.0)	17.4 (5.3)
Post	18.1 (6.4)	18.8 (3.6)	17.9 (4.7)
Word Discrimination in Noise Percent Correct:			
RE[2] Pre	65.3 (6.2)	60.7 (11.4)	69.5 (10.1)
Post	67.4 (6.6)	63.7 (15.8)	63.5 (18.0)
LE[3] Pre	63.2 (8.3)	58.8 (14.4)	67.3 (8.1)
Post	68.6 (7.3)	61.8 (16.5)	65.8 (12.1)
Standard Progressive Matrices Number Correct:			
Pre	25.7 (13.3)	28.8 (13.3)	28.8 (12.0)
Post	28.3 (14.4)	31.7 (12.2)	31.0 (9.6)

[1] in parentheses
[2] right ear
[3] left ear

following AIT. These improved scores were sometimes interpreted as indicative of AIT's effectiveness. However, the results of the SSW test in this study demonstrate that even without any treatment (control group), SSW number of errors decreased. The degree of improvement seen in the present study SSW results is similar to that described by Katz and Kram (1993) and ascribed to a learning effect. Furthermore, the behavioral test changes in the present study were seen over a period of only seven weeks, for each

of the three groups. Therefore, changes were most likely due to a practice/
learning effect, rather than a change in cognitive development.

For the Phonemic Synthesis Test, the mean number of items correct
increased by approximately .5 item for group C at the time of the seven-
week posttest. The mean number of items correct increased by approximately 2 for group E and P (Table 10.1). This degree of improvement is
consistent with results of Metzl (1969) for immediate retest using the Phonemic Synthesis. Therefore, a treatment effect is not suggested.

For the speech-in-noise test, the number correct increased by about 2
to 5 percent for groups E and P, for the right and left ears. The mean
speech-in-noise percentage correct for group C decreased by about 6 percent for the right ear and 1 percent for the left ear, as shown in Table
10.1.

Fisher's Auditory Problems Checklist
For the Fisher's Auditory Problems Checklist, the mean number of auditory behaviors indicated by parents as problems observed in their children decreased for each of the three groups at the time of posttest
compared to pretest. Parents of subjects in the placebo group noted the
greatest mean decrease (approximately three fewer items checked) in
problem behaviors (see Table 10.2).

Standard Progressive Matrices Test
The mean number of correct responses on the Standard Progressive
Matrices test increased slightly at the time of posttest (approximately 2
to 3 more correct of the 60 items administered) for each of the three
groups at posttest, as shown in Table 10.1. IQ, or visual reasoning, the
abilities measured by the Standard Progressive Matrices tests, would not
be expected to improve following stimulation via the auditory modality

**TABLE 10.2 Means and Standard Deviations[1] for the
Fisher's Auditory Problems Checklist**

Group	Experimental	Placebo	Control
Number of Items Checked by Parents:			
Pre	9.00	12.75	12.67
	(3.7)	(6.3)	(4.8)
Post	8.00	9.83	12.33
	(4.4)	(6.1)	(5.8)

[1] in parentheses

and surely not for the control group. Therefore, these results support a practice or learning effect.

Some degree of improvement was seen for the majority of the 10 behavioral tests or conditions over the seven-week period, regardless of treatment group. These results reveal important information for clinicians using a standard CAP battery to assess changes in auditory processing over time or following a therapy program. The results strongly suggest that the researcher or clinician should determine the degree of learning or practice effect for the tests administered before concluding that improvement has occurred based on a therapeutic intervention. If only one group had been examined in this study, or had a case study been carried out based on one of the children who showed improved performance, these results might have been erroneously interpreted as improvement in central auditory processing skills resulting from AIT treatment.

Pure-Tone Thresholds
Berard (1993) describes clinically significant differences between pure-tone thresholds at adjacent frequencies as indicators of deficient auditory processing. He reports that changes in thresholds following AIT eliminate these differences. In order to determine if evidence of such threshold changes could be found, changes in thresholds were compared between the three groups. Results indicated no statistically significant changes in threshold at 500, 1,000, 2,000 and 4,000 Hz, between groups at the .01 level of confidence. At the .05 level of confidence, pure-tone thresholds were significantly improved at 1,000 Hz and 2,000 Hz, for the left ear, for the placebo group, compared to the experimental group.

Electrophysiological Tests
For both the ABR and P3 recordings, each subject's right ear and left ear individual data points were compared. Statistically significant differences were not found between ears for any of the groups. Therefore, right and left ear data were combined for data analysis.

For the P3 response, difference waves were computed by subtracting the response to the frequent stimuli from the response to the infrequent stimuli, yielding a single wave to be analyzed for each trial. Both P3 amplitudes and latencies were determined based on the difference waves.

This study provided no physiological evidence that AIT has either a beneficial or a detrimental effect based on ABR latencies and interlatencies. In addition, there were no significant changes in P3 latencies or amplitudes between groups. Figures 10.2 and 10.3 show ABR and P3 recordings, respectively, from two subjects in the experimental group. These are representative of the recordings of subjects in each of the three groups.

**FIGURE 10.2   Replicated Auditory Brain Stem Response (ABR).
Recordings for one of the experimental group subjects before AIT
(top traces, ipsilateral recording; bottom traces, contralateral recordings; only the ipsilateral recordings were used in data analysis).
Traces are representative of recordings from subjects in each of the
three groups.**

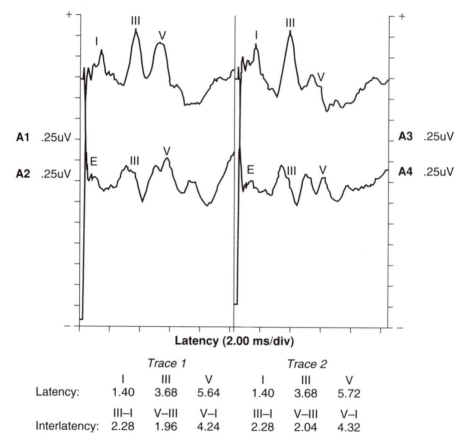

	Trace 1			*Trace 2*		
	I	III	V	I	III	V
Latency:	1.40	3.68	5.64	1.40	3.68	5.72
	III–I	V–III	V–I	III–I	V–III	V–I
Interlatency:	2.28	1.96	4.24	2.28	2.04	4.32

Auditory Brain Stem Response (ABR).   Pre- and posttest mean absolute and interwave latencies for the three CAPD groups are shown in
Table 10.3. In contrast to the general improvement on retest noted on the
behavioral tests, consistent changes were not found for ABR.

P3.   Analysis of P3 difference scores indicated that the mean P3 latency
decreased for group E and increased for group C, by nonsignificant

FIGURE 10.3   Replicated P3 Recordings for Experimental Subjects before AIT (top traces, frequent average; middle traces, infrequent average; bottom traces, difference waves). Traces are representative of recordings from subjects in each of the three groups.

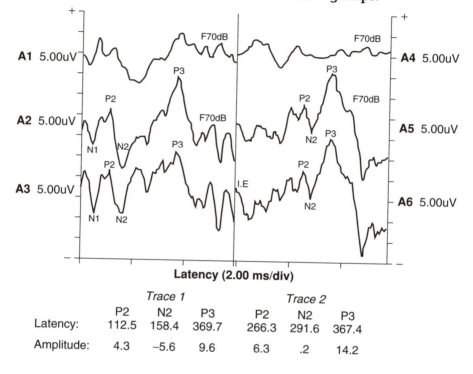

	Trace 1			Trace 2		
	P2	N2	P3	P2	N2	P3
Latency:	112.5	158.4	369.7	266.3	291.6	367.4
Amplitude:	4.3	−5.6	9.6	6.3	.2	14.2

degrees, and was essentially unchanged for the placebo group. Standard deviations were large, indicating a great deal of variability between subjects. Mean P3 amplitude increased for each of the three groups from pre- to posttest. Amplitude ratios (posttest divided by pretest) were calculated. Statistical analysis of the mean amplitude ratios, from 1.08 to 1.11 microvolts, indicated no significant P3 changes between groups. Table 10.3 shows the mean pre- and posttest values for P3 latency and amplitude for the three groups.

Comparison of This Study's Results to Other Published Research on AIT

Two studies of AIT were published over the past few years. Rimland and Edelson (1994) and Monville and Nelson (1994) suggested that AIT may

TABLE 10.3 Means and Standard Deviations[1] for the Electrophysiological Tests

Group		Experimental	Placebo	Control
ABR Latency (msec):				
Wave I	Pre	1.47 (.09)	1.58 (.20)	1.52 (.08)
	Post	1.49 (.18)	1.60 (.26)	1.51 (.11)
Wave III	Pre	3.64 (.11)	3.67 (.25)	3.61 (.16)
	Post	3.65 (.17)	3.63 (.23)	3.60 (.17)
Wave V	Pre	5.67 (.16)	5.56 (.23)	5.60 (.23)
	Post	5.64 (.19)	5.60 (.23)	5.59 (.21)
Wave I-III	Pre	2.17 (.09)	2.08 (.12)	2.08 (.15)
	Post	2.16 (.10)	2.04 (.15)	2.10 (.16)
Wave III-V	Pre	2.03 (.09)	1.90 (.19)	1.99 (.15)
	Post	1.99 (.08)	1.97 (.18)	1.99 (.13)
Wave I-V	Pre	4.20 (.13)	3.98 (.23)	4.07 (.19)
	Post	4.15 (.12)	3.97 (.22)	4.09 (.19)
P3 Latency (msec)				
	Pre	366 (78)	401 (51)	371 (124)
	Post	348 (53)	402 (80)	403 (66)
Amplitude (microvolts):				
	Pre	9.7 (2.4)	9.1 (1.8)	8.6 (1.7)
	Post	10.1 (2.4)	9.7 (2.0)	9.7 (1.8)

[1]in parentheses

be a beneficial treatment. This study, in contrast, does not support AIT as a beneficial treatment (at least for CAPD). However, there are considerable differences between studies in the populations examined and the measurements used.

Populations
A primary difference between the present study and that of Rimland and Edelson (1994) and Monville and Nelson (1994) is the population examined. The former studies reported positive results for the autistic population, a more severely impaired population compared to children with CAPD. There is no evidence that the two deficits, autism and CAPD, are closely related. However, based on Berard's (1993) writings, both types of problems are amenable to AIT.

Objectivity of Questionnaires
Another significant difference between the two published studies (Rimland & Edelson, 1994; Monville & Nelson, 1994) and the present one is that the changes reported in the two published studies were primarily based on parents' observations and responses to questionnaires. These may have been less objective than the behavioral and electrophysiological measures used in the present study.

Furthermore, parents of experimental subjects in the Rimland and Edelson (1994) study were aware that their children received AIT. Families had traveled long distances and paid their own travel and lodging expenses. Considering their expectations and expenditure of time and money, their objectivity could be questioned.

Parents in the Monville and Nelson study were surveyed after their children received AIT at their own expense. Responses were obtained from only 27 percent of families. Families that perceived benefit from AIT may have been more likely to respond than those who did not. Therefore, the sample might have been biased in favor of a positive response.

Control Group
An important strength of the present study was the control group, an admitted weakness of the Rimland and Edelson (1994) study. As a substitute, they used the control group ($n = 9$) from their pilot study (Rimland & Edelson, 1992) to compare with their experimental group ($n = 445$) treatment. They acknowledge this as a serious weakness in their large-scale study. This greatly limits the conclusions one can make about their AIT findings.

The present study was strengthened by matching subjects in the experimental, placebo, and control groups by age and SSW total number of errors. This type of matching procedure was not carried out for the

Rimland and Edelson study (1994) or the Monville and Nelson (1994) study. The disparate results between the present study and the Rimland and Edelson and the Monville and Nelson studies could be influenced by their lack of control subjects.

The control groups employed in the present study served to show the degree of practice or learning effect for the behavioral tests. A trend toward improved performance was seen on the behavioral CAP tests as well as the Fisher's Auditory Problems Checklist and the Standard Progressive Matrices test.

Had there been no control groups in the present study, it would have been easy to conclude that AIT improves central auditory processing abilities based on the improvement seen for the experimental group alone. This limitation may be common in studies based on patients in a standard clinical relationship (without a control group or adequate controls).

Research Finding No Benefit from AIT

A recent double-blind, placebo-controlled study (Zollweg et al., in press) reported results similar to that of the present study. The population assessed was individuals with mild to profound mental retardation, with autism, from 7 to 24 years of age. The Abberant Behavior Checklist was used to compare changes in behavior in a group that received AIT and a placebo group that received regular music. In addition, pure-tone thresholds were repeatedly measured for the two groups. Results indicated no significant differences in questionnaire responses (at one-, three-, and six-month periods) nor in pure-tone thresholds (at two-week and at three-, six-, and nine-month periods following AIT treatment) for the experimental versus the placebo group. The present study and the Zollweg and colleagues' study both implemented placebo/control groups, and each found that there was no benefit from AIT for the experimental group compared to the control group(s).

CONCLUSIONS

Recently, there has been a great deal of interest in therapeutic methods to remediate CAPD. Based on results of two published studies (Rimland & Edelson, 1994; Monville & Nelson, 1994), a number of unpublished studies, and a plethora of anecdotal reports, it was hoped that AIT might prove to be beneficial to children diagnosed with CAPD. Current knowledge of neural plasticity and of the possible benefits of increased stimulation to the auditory system suggest that a method that provides increased auditory stimulation could be of potential benefit. However, none of the behavioral or electrophysiological tests or the parental questionnaire results suggested that AIT improves central auditory processing skills or improves neural function in children with CAPD. The findings for children with CAPD are important because AIT is being administered at considerable cost in time and money to recipients (and AIT practitioners) throughout the United States.

ACKNOWLEDGMENTS

This study was a doctoral dissertation carried out at the State University of New York at Buffalo. I would like to gratefully acknowledge Dr. Steven Edelson's instruction on administering AIT and his advice on research methods and encouragement of this research on AIT. The Sertoma International, Western New York Chapters, donated funding for this project, as did members of the Parents' Information and Exchange (PIES) Group, Buffalo, New York. This project was partially funded by the Mark Diamond Research Fund (MDRF) grant from the State University of New York at Buffalo and the SSW Fund.

REFERENCES

American Speech-Language-Hearing Association (ASHA). (1989). Guidelines for screening for hearing impairment and middle ear disorders. *ASHA, 71–76.*
American Speech-Language-Hearing Association (ASHA). (1994). Auditory integration training (Ad Hoc Committee Report), *ASHA, 36*(11), 55–58.
Bannatyne, A. D., & Wichiarajote, P. (1969). Relationships between written spelling, motor functioning and sequencing skills. *Journal of Learning Disabilities, 2*(1), 6–18.
Baran, J. A., & Musiek, F. E. (1994). Behavioral assessment of the central auditory nervous system. In W. Rintelman (Ed.), *Hearing assessment.* Austin, TX: Pro-Ed.
Berard, G. (1993). *Hearing equals behavior* (Trans.). New Caanan, CT: Keats. (Original work published 1982).
BGC Enterprises, Inc. (1993). *Audio effects generator user's guide, Rev. B.* San Diego: Author.
Brandes, P., & Ehinger, D. (1981). The effects of early middle ear pathology on auditory perception and academic achievement. *Journal of Speech and Hearing Disorders, 46,* 301–307.
Butler, K. G. (1983). Language processing: Selective attention and mnemonic strategies. In E. Z. Lasky & J. Katz (Eds.), *Central auditory processing disorders: Problems of speech, language and learning* (pp. 297–315). Baltimore: University Park Press.

Campo, P., Subramaniam, M., & Henderson, D. (1991). Effect of conditioning exposures on hearing loss from traumatic exposure. *Hearing Research, 55,* 195–200.

Canlon, B., Borg, E., & Flock, A. (1988). Protection against noise trauma by pre-exposure to a low level acoustic stimulus. *Hearing Research, 34,* 197–200.

Canlon, B., Borg, E., & Lofstrand, P. (1992). Physiologic and morphologic aspects to low-level acoustic stimulation. In A. L. Dancer, D. Henderson, R. J. Salvi, & R. P. Hamernik (Eds.), *Noise-induced hearing loss* (pp. 489–499). New York: Mosby-Year Book.

Carhart, R., & Jerger, J. (1959). Preferred method for clinical determination of pure-tone thresholds. In I. M. Ventry, J. B. Chaiklin, & R. F. Dixon (Eds.), *Hearing measurement: A book of readings* (pp. 96–108). New York: Appleton-Century-Crofts.

Evans, W., Webster, D., & Cullen, J. (1983). Auditory brainstem responses in neonatally sound deprived CBA/J mice. *Hearing Research, 10,* 269–277.

Ferre, J., & Wilber, L. A. (1986). Normal and learning disabled children's auditory processing skills. An experimental test battery. *Ear and Hearing, 7,* 336–343.

Fisher, L. (1980). *Fisher's Auditory Problems Checklist.* Cedar Rapids, IA: Grant Woods Area Education Agency.

Flynn, P. T., & Byrne, M. C. (1970). Relationship between reading and selected auditory abilities of third-grade children. *Journal of Speech Hearing Research, 13,* 731–740.

Folsom, R., Weber, B., & Thompson, G. (1983). Auditory brainstem responses in children with early recurrent middle ear disease. *Annals of Otology Rhinology and Laryngology, 92,* 249–253.

Howard, M. R., & Hulit, L. M. (1992). Response patterns to central auditory tests and the clinical evaluation of language fundamentals-revised: A pilot study. *Perceptual and Motor Skills, 74,* 120–122.

Huttenlocher, P. R. (1990). Morphometric study of human cerebral cortex development. *Neuropsychologia, 28*(6), 517–527.

Ivey, R. G. (1992). The P300 response in children. *The Hearing Journal, 45*(10), 27–32.

Ivey, R. G., & Willeford, J. A. (1988). Three tests of CNS auditory function. *Human Communication in Canada, 12*(3), 35–43.

Jerger, S., Jerger, J., Alford, B., & Abrams, S. (1983). Development of speech intelligibility in children with recurrent otitis media. *Ear and Hearing, 4,* 138–145.

Jerger, S., Martin, R. C., & Jerger, J. (1987). Specific auditory perceptual dysfunction in a learning disabled child. *Ear and Hearing, 8,* 78– 86.

Jirsa, R. E. (1992). The clinical utility of the P3 AERP in children with auditory processing disorders. *Journal of Speech and Hearing Research, 35,* 903–912.

Jirsa, R. E., & Clontz, K. B. (1990). Long latency auditory event-related potentials from children with auditory processing disorders. *Ear and Hearing, 11*(3), 222–232.

Johnson, D. W., Enfield, M. L., & Sherman, R. E. (1981). The use of the staggered spondaic word and the competing environmental sounds tests in the evaluation of central auditory function of learning disabled children. *Ear and Hearing, 2*(2), 70–77.

Katz, J. (1983). Phonemic synthesis. In E. Z. Lasky & J. Katz (Eds.), *Central auditory processing disorders: Problems of speech, language, and learning* (pp. 269–295). Austin, TX: Pro-Ed.

Katz, J. (1987). *SSW workshop manual*. Unpublished.

Katz, J. (1992). Classification of central auditory processing disorders. In J. Katz, N. A. Stecker, & D. Henderson (Eds.), *Central auditory processing: A transdisciplinary view* (pp. 81–91). Boston: Mosby-Year Book.

Katz, J., & Burge, C. (1971). Auditory perception training for children with learning disabilities. *Menorah Medical Journal, 2,* 18–29.

Katz, J., & Cohen, C. F. (1985). Auditory training for children with perceptual difficulties. *Journal of Childhood Communication Disorders, 9,* 65–81.

Katz, J., & Harmon, C. H. (1982). *Phonemic synthesis: Blending sounds into words.* Allen, TX: Developmental Learning Materials.

Katz, J., & Illmer, R. (1972). Auditory perception in children with learning disabilities. In J. Katz (Ed.), *Handbook of clinical audiology* (4th ed.) (pp. 239–255). Baltimore: Williams and Wilkins.

Katz, J., & Kram, J. (1993, November). Test-retest of the SSW in learning disabled children. *SSW Reports,* pp. 1–3.

Katz, J., & Medol, I. (1972). The use of phonemic synthesis in speech therapy. *Menorah Medical Journal, 3,* 10–18.

Katz, J., & Wilde, L. (1985). Auditory processing disorders. In J. Katz (Ed.), *Handbook of clinical audiology* (3rd ed.) (pp. 664–688). Baltimore: Williams and Wilkins.

Keller, W. D. (1992). Auditory processing disorder or attention-deficit disorder? In J. Katz, N. A. Stecker, & D. Henderson (Eds.), *Central auditory processing: A transdisciplinary view* (pp. 107–114). Boston: Mosby-Year Book.

Kraus, N., McGee, T., Ferre, J., Hoeppner, J., Carrell, T., Sharma, A., & Nicol, T. (1993). Mismatch negativity in the neurophysiologic/behavioral evaluation of auditory processing deficits: A case study. *Ear and Hearing, 14*(4), 223–234.

Lenhardt, M. (1981). Childhood central auditory processing disorder with brainstem evoked response verification. *Archives Otolaryngology, 107,* 623– 625.

Merzenich, M. M., Jenkins, W. M., Johnston, P., Schreiner, C., Miller, S. L., & Tallal, P. (1996). Temporal processing deficits of language-impaired children ameliorated by training. *Science, 271,* 77–80.

Metzl, M. N. (1969). *Measurements of sound synthesis ability in second, fourth, and sixth grade children and adults* Unpublished masters' thesis. Hunter College, New York.

Milgram, N. W., MacLeod, C. M., & Petit, T. L. (1987). Neuroplasticity, learning and memory. In N. W. Milgram, C. M. MacLeod, & T. L. Petit, (Eds.), *Neuroplasticity, learning and memory: Proceedings of a symposium held at the University of Toronto, Scarborough, Ontario, March 25, 1986* (pp. 1–16). New York: Alan R. Liss.

Monville, D. K., & Nelson, N. W. (1994). Parental viewpoints on change following auditory integration training for autism. *American Journal of Speech-Language Pathology, 3*(2), 41–51.

Mulder, R. L., & Curtin, J. (1955). Vocal phonic ability and silent reading achievement. *Elementary School Journal, 56,* 121–123.

Musiek, F. E., & Baran, J. A. (1986). Neuroanatomy, neurophysiology, and central auditory assessment. Part I. Brain stem. *Ear and Hearing, 7*(4), 207–219.

Musiek, F. E., Geurkink, N. A., & Kietal, S. A. (1982). Test battery assessment of auditory perceptual dysfunction in children. *Laryngoscope, 92,* 251–257.

Nast, K. A. (1992). *Suprathreshold changes associated with noise-induced resistance to noise-induced hearing loss (NIHL).* Unpublished master's thesis, State University of New York at Buffalo.

Paden, E., Matthies, M., & Novak, M. (1989). Recovery from OME-related phonologic delay following tube placement. *Journal of Speech and Hearing Disorders, 54,* 94–100.

Paden, E., Novak, M., & Beiter, A. (1987). Predictors of phonologic inadequacy in young children prone to otitis media. *Journal of Speech Hearing Disorders, 52,* 232–242.

Pinheiro, M. (1977). Tests of central auditory function in children with learning disabilities. In R. W. Keith (Ed.), *Central auditory dysfunction* (pp. 223–256). New York: Grune and Stratton.

Polich, J. (1993). P300 in clinical applications: Meaning, method, and measurement. In E. Niedermeyer & F. Lopes de Silva (Eds.), *Electroencephalography: Basic principles, clinical applications, and related fields* (3rd ed.) (pp. 1005–1018). Baltimore: Williams and Wilkins.

Raven, J. C. (1990). *Standard Progressive Matrices Test.* Oxford, England: Oxford Psychologists Press. (Originally published 1936).

Raven, J. C., Court, J. H., & Raven, J. (1985). *A manual for Raven's Progressive Matrices and Vocabulary Scales.* London: H. K. Lewis.

Rimland, B., & Edelson, S. (1992). Auditory integration training in autism: A pilot study. *Autism Research Institute Publication No. 112.* (Available from the Autism Research Institute, 4182 Adams Avenue, San Diego, CA 92116.)

Rimland, B., & Edelson, S. (1994). The effects of auditory integration training on autism. *American Journal of Speech Language Pathology, 3*(2), 16–24.

Roberts, J., Burchinal, M., & Koch, M. (1988). Otitis media in early childhood and its relationship to later phonological development. *Journal of Speech and Hearing Disorders, 53,* 424–432.

Robertson, D., & Irvine, D. R. F. (1989). Plasticity of frequency organization in auditory cortex of guinea pigs with partial unilateral deafness. *The Journal of Comparative Neurology, 282,* 456–471.

Rosensweig, M. R. (1984). Experience, memory and the brain. *American Psychologist, 39,* 365–376.

Ryals, B. M., Rubel, E. W., & Lippe, W. (1991). Issues in neural plasticity as related to cochlear implants in children. *American Journal of Otology, 12*(suppl.), 22–27.

Sayers, B. McA., Beagley, H. A., & Henshall, W. R. (1974). Mechanism of auditory evoked responses. *Nature, 247,* 481–483.

Schneider, D. (1992). Audiologic management of central auditory processing disorders. In J. Katz, N. Stecker, & D. Henderson (Eds.), *Central auditory processing: A transdisciplinary view* (pp. 161–168). Boston: Mosby-Year Book.

Sloan, C. (1980). Auditory processing disorders and language development. In P. Levenson & C. Sloan (Eds.), *Auditory processing and language: Clinical and research perspectives* (pp. 101–116). New York: Grune and Stratton.

Tallal, P., Miller, S. L., Bedi, G., Byma, G., Wang, X., Nagarajan, S. S., Schreiner, C., Jenkins, W. M., & Merzenich, M. M. (1996). Language comprehension in language-learning impaired children improved with acoustically modified speech. *Science, 271,* 81–84.

Tillery, K. L. (1992). *Central auditory processing abilities of attention deficit hyperactivity disordered children: With and without methylphenidate.* Unpublished master's thesis. Illinois State University, Normal, IL.

Webster, D. B. (1974). Audition. In E. C. Carterette & M. P. Friedman (Eds.), *Handbook of perception, Vol 3: Biology of perceptual systems* (pp. 449–482). New York: Academic Press.

Webster, D. B. (1983). Auditory neuronal sizes after a unilateral conductive hearing loss. *Experimental Neurology, 79,* 130–140.

Webster, D. B., & Webster, M. (1977). Neonatal sound deprivation affects brain stem auditory nuclei. *Archives Otolaryngology, 103,* 392–396.

Webster, D. B., & Webster, M. (1978). Cochlear nerve projections following organ of Corti destruction. *Otolaryngology, 86,* 342–353.

Webster, D. B., & Webster, M. (1979). Effects of neonatal conductive hearing loss on brain stem auditory nuclei. *Annals of Otology, 88,* 684–688.

Welsh, L. W., Welsh, J. J., & Healy, M. P. (1983). Effect of sound deprivation on central hearing. *Laryngoscope, 93,* 1569–1575.

Willeford, J. A., & Burleigh, J. M. (1985). *Handbook of central auditory processing disorders in children.* New York: Grune and Stratton.

Witkin, B. R. (1971). Auditory perception-implications for language development. *Language Speech Hearing Services in Schools, 2*(4), 31–52.

Woods, B. T., & Teuber, H. L. (1978). Changing patterns of childhood aphasia. *Annals of Neurology, 3,* 273–280.

Young, M. L. (1983). Neuroscience, pragmatic competence and auditory processing. In E. Z. Lasky & J. Katz (Eds.), *Central auditory processing disorders: Problems of speech, language and learning* (pp. 141–162). Baltimore: University Park Press.

Zollweg, W., Vance, V., & Palm, D. (in press). A double-blind, placebo controlled study of the efficacy of auditory integration training. *American Journal of Audiology.*

11

CENTRAL AUDITORY PROCESSING ASSESSMENT AND THERAPEUTIC STRATEGIES FOR CHILDREN WITH ATTENTION DEFICIT HYPERACTIVITY DISORDER

KIM L. TILLERY
State University of New York at Fredonia

The 1990s should be referred to as "the awareness decade," considering professionals are educating themselves and others more than at any other time in history. This is particularly true in understanding the symptoms of illness and disorders, improving assessment techniques, and implementing new therapy procedures. Awareness has increased dramatically for both attention deficit hyperactivity disorder (ADHD) and for central auditory processing disorder (CAPD). Barkley (1990) points out that ADHD is the most common childhood disorder. CAPD is another common problem and these two disorders are often diagnosed in the same children.

Before discussing central auditory processing (CAP) evaluation and remediation strategies for those who have ADHD, it may be beneficial to enhance the reader's awareness of what it is like to have an auditory processing disorder. CAPD refers to the inability to utilize effectively what one hears (Katz, 1992). Imagine a child in a kindergarten class or in first grade who exhibits a phonemic decoding type of CAPD. This individual often misunderstands what is said, substitutes similar sounds, requires a longer than normal period of time to respond, has a word finding difficulty, and has weak receptive language skills (Katz, 1992).

Imagine the following scenario in a classroom where the teacher says to the students:

> "Good morning, class. I am going to read a story to you about *Goldilocks and the Three Bears.*"

> > Once upon a time there were three bears who lived in a little cottage. One day while eating breakfast, the papa bear said, "My porridge is too hot." The mama bear said, "My porridge is too cold," and the baby bear said, "Yes, but my porridge is just right."

As the story is read to the class, this child with a decoding CAPD misunderstands the story and hears:

> "Good Morning, class. I lill read a story to you called *Boldirocks and Gatree Pears.*"

> > Once open a chime, dare were tree pears who rivved in a widdle gotitch. Sunday when eating feckers, the bapa pear said, "My marbridge is too hot." The nana pear said, "My marbridge is too old," and the baby pear said, "Yes, but my marbridge is chuck light."

Imagine the frustration a child with a decoding CAPD experiences when presented with new and complex auditory information, particularly when spoken quickly. This child is surprised that her classmates were smiling when the story was read to them, as she misunderstands most of the story and becomes quite anxious. She remembers from previous experience that the teacher asks questions about a story after reading it. The child knows that she is unable to answer the questions correctly, because she did not understand the story.

This illustration becomes more complex with the realization that the child may also have characteristics of ADHD. Imagine how meaningless the story becomes if there are distractions in class and the child's attention is drawn away at several points, causing her to miss the information. Professionals often question whether the child has difficulty processing the auditory information, due to a CAPD, or if a CAP test failure is related to the child's attention impairment. Obviously, if an individual is unable to attend to auditory information, then the information will not be responded to properly; however, if an individual is attentive, but still does not effectively process the auditory message, then CAPD may be the problem.

CONTROLLING TEST BEHAVIOR

Commonly, children with ADHD are more attentive in a novel or one-to-one situation (Barkley, 1990). Even though a test session meets these criteria, the individual with ADHD may become distracted and less attentive during a one- to two-hour evaluation. It may be necessary to employ specific measures, such as the following, to assist in maintaining the client's attention.

1. A simple measure that aids attention is to provide breaks between tests. Usually, the child will be grateful to remove the earphones and to receive a few minutes to relax. A child who refuses the break should be encouraged to step out of the booth, take a walk, or get a drink of water.
2. During a test procedure, a clinician will enhance the child's attention by giving positive reinforcements to indicate the child is doing a good job. This may be done with smiles, head nods, verbal praise, and even clapping hands to show that the response was particularly good.
3. Another maneuver that maintains the child's attention is to provide an alternate response mode, as the child with ADHD will probably become less attentive on the second-test ear. For example, asking the child to state how many beeps he hears (instead of hand raising when the tone is heard) may enhance his attention, as the task is now to listen for the one, two, or three beeps.
4. When the child responds to the carrier phrase, "Are you ready?" with "Yes. I am ready," and therefore obliterates the test stimulus, the clinician should stop the test tape, instruct the child not to talk when the test question is provided and proceed. The child who talks excessively during the evaluation may need to be reinstructed several times that the unnecessary vocal responses will interfere with his hearing the stimuli. Reliable results are unattainable when a child does not attend or talks during the presentation of the stimuli. By stopping the test tape, the clinician can assist the child who is impulsive, hyperactive, and/or distractible.
5. Probably the simplest solution to assist with the attention of a child with ADHD, during CAPD assessment, is to schedule the evaluation while the child is under the influence of his central nervous system (CNS) stimulant medication. Individuals with ADHD usually receive a CNS medication as part of their multimodal treatment for the ADHD (Barkley, 1990).

EFFECT OF MEDICATION ON
ADHD BEHAVIOR AND CAP TESTS

In the 1970s, there were over 2,000 studies that indicated that the CNS stimulant medication, particularly Ritalin, enhances the attention of children with ADHD (Barkley, 1990). Currently, there are five known studies that investigated the effects of Ritalin on the CAP test performance of children with ADHD. These studies have conflicting results.

Three of the studies (Keith & Engineer, 1991; Gascon, Johnson, & Burd, 1986; Cook et al.,1993) found significant improvement in test performance of children with ADHD when medicated with their CNS stimulant medication. Another study (Ivey & Jerome, 1988) found no significant improvement in the overall CAP test performance when the children were medicated verses nonmedicated. The fifth study (Tillery, 1992) found significant improvement on two of the nine test variables. The left ear Dichotic Digit (DD) and Staggered Spondaic Word (SSW) reversal measures were improved when the children were evaluated when medicated with their normal dosage of Ritalin. The conflicting results possibly stem from (1) the variety of criteria utilized to select the subjects with ADHD, (2) the various CAP tests employed in the studies, and (3) not controlling for learning (e.g., whether all the subjects were first evaluated when nonmedicated and then were evaluated in a medicated condition for the second test session.

There is a paucity of evidence as to the effectiveness of CNS stimulant medication on the CAP abilities of those with ADHD. A child with ADHD generally receives medication to assist in attending, especially during the school day. Therefore, it may also assist the child in attending during a lengthy evaluation.

DIFFERENTIAL DIAGNOSIS OF ADHD AND CAPD

Because of the widespread awareness of ADHD, it is more likely that those who have ADHD will have this diagnosis before receiving a CAP evaluation. However, a child may be referred for an auditory processing evaluation because of symptoms that are associated with either CAPD or ADHD (Keller, 1992). When a clinician provides differential diagnostic assessment, there are procedures that can assist in obtaining reliable test results in children who have symptoms of ADHD.

A child who is referred probably exhibits some degree of inattentiveness and distractibility. When a child fails two of four CAP tests, at 4:00 in the afternoon, a professional should question whether the performance is a true indication of the child's auditory processing abilities or if the test scores were influenced by fatigue from the long school day. Failure on CAP tests in a morning evaluation likely identifies CAP difficulties without the influence of fatigue.

Keith (1994) recommended an approach for assisting with differential diagnosis of a child with possible ADHD and/or CAPD by use of the Auditory Continuous Performance Test (ACPT). The ACPT is a vigilance measure that evaluates the child's auditory attention and impulsivity. The child is instructed to raise his thumb when he hears the target word *dog.* Six sets of 90 words in each set are presented. If the child does not raise his thumb when he hears the word *dog,* then an attentive impairment may exist. If the child raises his thumb to words other than the target word, he is demonstrating impulsivity. The child's performance on the first set of words may be compared to the performance on the sixth set of words, to investigate performance over time.

The child should be instructed to raise his thumb, and not to push a button that is commonly found in the audiologist's sound booth. A child may appear to be more impulsive if told to push the button, because this response mode will likely increase the impulsivity of almost any child.

Another aid in differential diagnosis is a parent and/or teacher questionnaire, which provides a checklist of behaviors commonly associated with ADHD and CAPD (see Appendix A). The observed behaviors are dispersed throughout the questionnaire, and a heading of *CAPD/ADHD Questionnaire* may be omitted to prevent rater bias. Based on the responses, the clinician can explain to the parent that the child manifests common behaviors seen among individuals with ADHD, CAPD, or both disorders, enabling an appropriate referral.

CASE STUDIES

The following two case studies illustrate assessment and remediation strategies for children with CAPD and ADHD.

Case Study 1

The first unique case involves an 11-year-old male, named Joshua, who was diagnosed with ADHD at age 7. He was receiving tutoring, counseling, and behavioral intervention, together with Ritalin medication for treatment of ADHD. Joshua performed two years below grade level in reading, displayed difficulty in understanding new concepts, and was weak in spelling skills.

The school nurse referred Joshua for a complete audiological evaluation because of an apparent bilateral hearing loss suggested by the hearing screening (see Figure 11.1). Two years earlier, Joshua also demonstrated a profound loss in the left ear and a mild loss in the right ear (see Figure 11.2). At that time, auditory brain stem response (ABR) measurements suggested normal hearing, bilaterally. It was unclear why Joshua was displaying possible nonorganic behavior for the past two years.

On the current evaluation, Joshua displayed poor hearing thresholds for each ear (see Figure 11.3), but normal (Type A) tympanograms and normal levels for ipsilateral and contralateral acoustic reflex thresholds. The clinician observed Joshua's difficulty in understanding directions and his slow manner in responding to the stimuli, which are characteristic of auditory processing dysfunction. Another sign frequently observed

FIGURE 11.1   Joshua's Hearing Thresholds from His School Screening Test

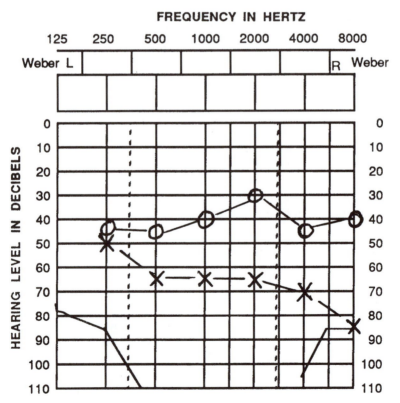

FIGURE 11.2   Joshua's Hearing Thresholds, Two Years Prior to the School Screening Test

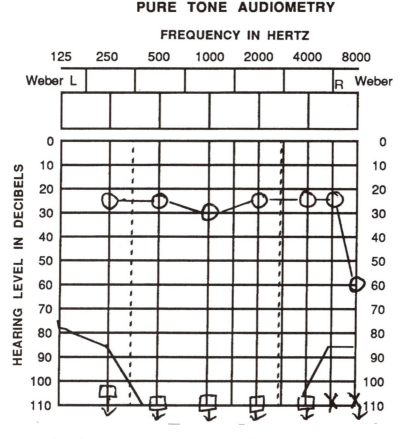

was Joshua's speech reception thresholds (SRTs) were better than his pure-tone thresholds (PTAs). This is a common sign of both nonorganic and CAPD cases (Katz, 1992).

The oral response of the SRT requires the client to understand and repeat the presented spondaic words. To investigate the possibility that Joshua's SRTs might improve, the test was repeated using a pointing response to the picture of the target word. Under these conditions, the SRTs improved from 25 dB HL to10 dB HL for the right ear and from 15 dB HL to 5 dB HL for the left ear. The clinician speculated that Joshua's SRTs improved because the language requirement for repeating the target words was removed from the task.

The combination of Joshua's (1) slow responses, (2) difficulty in understanding directions, and (3) improved SRTs when oral language

FIGURE 11.3   Joshua's Hearing Thresholds, Obtained One Month after the School Screening Test

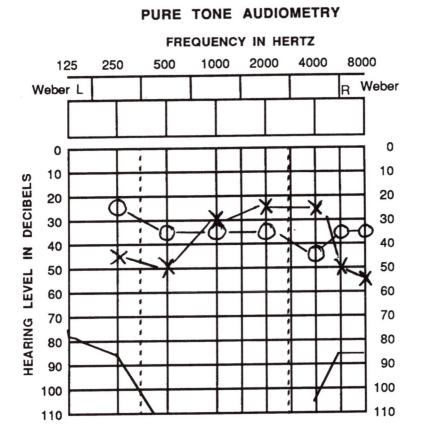

was not required suggested the possibility that Joshua might have a central auditory dysfunction. Furthermore, children such as Joshua who have ADHD may be at risk for a CAPD (Tillery, 1992).

Joshua returned the following week for a CAP evaluation, scheduled in the morning to control for fatigue, while he was under the influence of his Ritalin medication, to control for attention. Another important consideration when evaluating children with ADHD is motivation. To enhance Joshua's motivation, the clinician informed Joshua that after he completed the evaluation, he would receive an entire roll of stickers as a reward for his high level of concentration. Joshua smiled at the opportunity of leaving the office with about 400 stickers.

The peripheral hearing assessment indicated PTAs of 15 dB HL and 20 dB HL for the right and left ears, respectively (see Figure 11.4). Joshua

FIGURE 11.4 Joshua's Obtained Audiometric Test Results, Prior to the CAP Evaluation

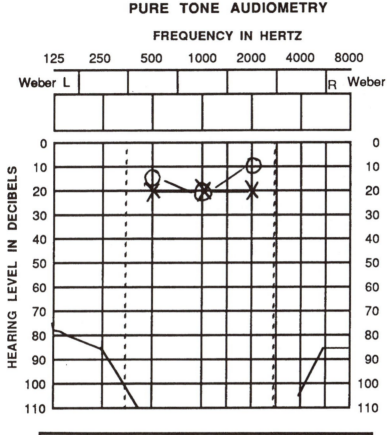

was encouraged to remove the earphones and step out of the sound booth prior to obtaining SRTs of 5 dB HL for the right ear and 10 dB HL for the left ear. Another break was provided to Joshua before the word discrimination measurements. He obtained scores of 92 percent for the left ear and 76 percent for the right ear, which was below normal limits, suggesting a possible decoding type of CAPD.

After another break, a battery of central auditory processing tests was administered to assess Joshua's ability to deal with less redundant information. Joshua's test performance suggested both decoding and integration CAP problems. The following recommendations were given:

1. Preferential seating is important for Joshua so that he can benefit from both acoustic and visual cues in class. A distance of 6 to 10 feet from the teacher/speaker is considered most beneficial. The recommendation was to have Joshua sit in the second row to enhance visual cues from other strong students seated in front and beside him.

When a teacher gives rapid directions, such as "Take out your math book, turn to page 10, do problems one through six, but skip seven, eight and nine and then do the rest of the problems," Joshua may have more success in responding to these lengthy directions if he is able to look at the students in front of him or beside him for visual cues. A child with ADHD who sits in the front row may turn around for visual cues from the child seated behind him. The teacher may regard this as a child who is not paying attention, when in fact it is a child who needs to compensate for a CAP problem.

2. Joshua's teachers should be aware that he may have difficulty in understanding what is asked of him, and he may forget lengthy information presented to him, especially when the auditory message is rapid. This problem could cause him to miss important verbal information and become frustrated. Joshua should be encouraged to ask for repeated directions, when necessary, and be provided extra time to respond, if needed. Directions stated in shorter sentences or phrases generally help these children.

3. Because of poor decoding, Joshua will likely benefit from receiving auditory processing therapy that targets strengthening his phonemic knowledge of vowel and consonant sounds, and grammatical morphemes. Such therapy may include the Phonemic Synthesis (PS) Training program (Katz & Fletcher, 1982).

Joshua exhibited difficulty in differentiating vowel sounds, which is a classic problem seen in individuals with CAP decoding problems. Upon completion of the PS training program, Joshua should be exposed to the Auditory Discrimination in Depth (ADD) program (Lindamood & Lindamood, 1969). The ADD program compliments the PS program by providing targets to assist in the discrimination of vowel sounds. Exposure to these therapy programs will typically improve reading and spelling skills.

4. Joshua may benefit from receiving visual-rhyming therapy to increase his ability to integrate auditory and visual information. Appendix B provides the details of this therapy that incorporates Joshua's weekly spelling words.

5. Joshua should receive a CAP reevaluation in one year to ascertain the effects of maturation and therapeutic strategies.

6. Children with ADHD frequently complain of noise intolerance but may not be found to display a speech-in-noise disability on audiological testing, as in Joshua's case. Thus, this may not be part of Joshua's CAPD, but rather a characteristic of ADHD. Nevertheless, it requires consideration. Joshua may benefit from wearing noise protection devices (earplugs) when in noisy listening situations, (especially when it is unnecessary to hear an auditory message). Examples of such situations include when studying at home, on the school bus, in the cafeteria, and when taking tests.

Case Study 2

Rob was 6 years old when he was diagnosed with ADHD, and at age 9, he was found to have a CAPD, primarily in decoding and secondarily in tolerance-fading memory (TFM). He had been receiving occupational therapy twice a week to improve his fine motor skills and tutoring assistance in reading once a week. His spelling and reading skills were about two years below grade level.

Rob also had two 50-minute auditory therapy sessions per week for nine weeks. For all 18 sessions, he received two phonemic synthesis training lessons, visual-rhyming therapy, speech reading, and instruction in manipulation of listening environments. He was motivated and never hesitated to perform his best. Rob came to therapy sessions after the school day and was usually fatigued, but he took a nap on the trip to the clinic.

Pre- and posttherapy test measures are displayed in Table 11.1, with both quantitative and qualitative results. *Quantitative* results are the percentage score for correct responses, whereas *qualitative* results are the number of correct responses without any form of struggle. For the staggered spondaic word (SSW) test, quantitative (raw percent error) test results are provided for four measures: right competing, left competing, right noncompeting, and left noncompeting. The clinician also observed

TABLE 11.1   Rob's Pre- and Posttherapy Test Results on the Staggered Spondaic Word (SSW), Phonemic Synthesis (PS), and Speech-in-Noise (S/N) Tests. Qualitative scoring permits an error to be recorded if it shows significant difficulty in responding normally, even if the eventual response is correct.

		RNC	RC	LC	LNC	Delays
SSW	Pre:	2	6	10	3	42
	Post:	1	3	5	2	13

PS	Pre:	Quantitative-	18 correct
		Qualitative-	6 correct
			9 quiet rehearsals
			4 nonfusions
			4 delays
	Post:	Quantitative-	21 correct
		Qualitative-	18 correct
			0 quiet rehearsals
			0 nonfusions
			3 delays

S/N

		Quiet	*Noise*	*Difference Score*
	Pre:			
	RE	92%	48%	44%
	LE	76%	40%	36%
	Post:			
	RE	96%	48%	48%
	LE	92%	40%	52%

for qualitative responses, such as quick or delayed response manner, perseverations, smushes, tongue twisters, or stating "Are you ready?" or "Yes" to the SSW carrier phrase (Katz, 1992); however, only delayed responses were noted. For the Phonemic Synthesis (PS) test, both quantitative and qualitative information may be obtained, as provided on the PS test form.

The clinician who observes the child's displayed struggle (qualitative score) in producing the proper responses may infer specific difficulties. A child who produces 42 delays in a test environment, for instance, undoubtedly experiences delays in the classroom.

Rob's pretherapy test scores indicated auditory processing dysfunction, but his qualitative struggle with 42 delays on the SSW test and several on the PS test (9 quiet rehearsals, 4 nonfusions, and 4 delays) were also taken into account. Upon completion of nine weeks of therapy, Rob displayed only 13 delays on the SSW test and three delays on the PS test.

Frequently, during the initial therapy lessons, Rob looked to the clinician for a sign that indicated he correctly responded. After the eighth lesson of the PS training, he became more confident in knowing that his responses were indeed correct, and rarely looked to the clinician for feedback. Further, he began to provide the proper responses without any form of struggle, which was also evident on the posttherapy measures.

Another important consideration when providing phonemic awareness therapy is to be aware that the individual's poor word discrimination score may well improve, thus an ear with normal speech-in-noise ability on pretesting may actually be revealed as having a speech-in-noise problem after receiving CAP therapy. Rob displayed a 76 percent word discrimination score on pretherapy testing, which improved to 92 percent on posttherapy. His speech-in-noise scores were unchanged, indicating more of a speech-in-noise problem in his right ear than was previously thought.

It is possible that Rob's auditory processing dysfunction would not have appeared extreme, if his noted delays and other qualitative struggles were not observed, as his quantitative scores were borderline CAP. A child who demonstrates many delays in responding to auditory information often experiences frustration, fatigue, and confusion in academic subjects. Rob's expressed and noted fatigue at the end of his school day is common among those children who exert a high concentration level to effectively utilize the auditory message. Rob improved significantly in providing proper responses, and did so without the immense struggle seen initially.

In addition to the pre- and initial posttest scores, Rob received another CAP evaluation 18 months after therapy. It revealed no evidence of CAP dysfunction on the SSW or PS tests (see Table 11.2) but did show a mild bilateral speech-in-noise problem. Rob's mother reports that Rob's spelling and reading skills are at grade level and that he enjoys writing stories.

SUMMARY

Reliably evaluating the CAPD abilities of children with ADHD may be a challenge, but it is not impossible when the clinician is aware of strategies that enhance the attentive ability of children with this disorder. These strategies may also assist the child's inattentiveness during auditory processing therapy. Therapeutic measures of CAPD should be implemented according to the type of auditory processing problem that is found. Thus, the clinician should be aware of (1) the particular types of

TABLE 11.2 Rob's Test Results, 18 Months Posttherapy, on the Staggered Spondaic Word (SSW), Phonemic Synthesis (PS), and Speech-in-Noise (S/N) Tests. Qualitative scoring permits an error to be recorded if it shows significant difficulty in responding normally, even if the eventual response is correct.

		RNC	RC	LC	LNC	Delays
SSW		0	2	2	0	7
PS		Quantitative-	23 correct			
		Qualitative-	23 correct			
			1 quiet rehearsal			
			0 nonfusions			
			1 delay			
S/N						

		Quiet	*Noise*	*Difference Score*
	RE	96%	64%	32%
	LE	100%	60%	40%

CAPD, (2) the specific therapy strategies that remediate these difficulties, and (3) the fact that progress may be better understood using both quantitative and qualitative measures. The overall objective is for therapy to aid individuals with their auditory processing, while minimizing their ADHD behaviors.

APPENDIX A: CAPD/ADHD QUESTIONNAIRE

Name _____ Date _____

D.O.B. _____ Grade _____ School _____

Physician _____ Insurance _____

Please check the following behaviors that may be pertinent to this child. Circle the option that applies to the child, for questions that provide multiple choices.

Observer: _____

Medical History

_____ 1. History of hearing loss

_____ 2. History of ear infections

_____ 3. Pre- or perinatal complications (e.g., low birth weight, hypoxia, head trauma, high fever, Rh incompatibility, seizures, jaundice, etc.)

_____ 4. History of allergies, asthma, reactive airway disease (RAD), frequent colds and upper respiratory infections

_____ 5. History of hypo/ hyperactivity

_____ 6. History of attention deficit hyperactivity disorder (ADHD). If so:

   a) At what age was your child diagnosed? _____

   b) Diagnosed by _____ Profession _____

   c) Is your child receiving medication for ADHD? _____

   d) How long does it take to see the medication's effect? _____

   e) Is your child receiving

      counseling _____

      tutoring _____

      behavioral intervention _____

_____ 7. Has your child or a family member been diagnosed with a learning disorder?

_____ 8. Has any other family member been diagnosed with ADHD or CAPD?

Listening Skills

_____ 1. Says "Huh?" or "What?" frequently

_____ 2. At times, appears to have a hearing loss

_____ 3. Frequently asks for directions to be repeated

_____ 4. Responds in a slow or delayed manner when spoken to

_____ 5. Responds too quickly to situations without waiting for instructions

_____ 6. Misunderstands what is said most of the time

_____ 7. Appears as if he/she is not paying attention

_____ 8. Exhibits a low tolerance for noise

_____ 9. Is easily distracted in noisy situations

_____10. Shows enhanced communication when visual information is provided with audition

_____11. Displays some/extreme difficulty when provided with lengthy/complex information

_____12. Has difficulty in understanding speech sounds

_____13. Does not understand the verbal message, especially in background noise

_____14. Often "hears" a similar word (*bath* vs. *math*)

_____15. Shows difficulty in differentiating musical instruments or notes

Academic Skills

_____ 1. Displays inconsistency in school performance

_____ 2. Rushes through homework or classroom work without realizing that errors were made

_____ 3. Is unmotivated to learn new concepts

_____ 4. Reveals better *performance* results than *verbal* results on tests

_____ 5. Performs well in a one-to-one situation

_____ 6. Is disruptive in class

_____ 7. Interrupts peers or teacher

_____ 8. Improves in performance when in a structured environment

_____ 9. Displays weak reading/writing or spelling skills

_____10. Has difficulty explaining a story or idea

_____11. Does not complete tasks or is not organized with tasks

_____12. Appears unusually fatigued toward the end of the school day

Additional

_____ 1. (Requires/required) articulation therapy

_____ 2. (Requires/ required) language therapy

_____ 3. Seems to enjoy novel situations

_____ 4. Has difficulty in taking turns

_____ 5. Fidgets with hands or feet

_____ 6. Appears forgetful during daily routines

_____ 7. Loses items necessary to complete daily activities

_____ 8. Remembers final directions better than initial directions

_____ 9. Exerts more concentration than usual

_____10. Reverses letters or sounds when writing or speaking

_____11. Is poor at drawing geometrical shapes

The following information should not be displayed on the questionnaire:

1. The heading may be omitted to prevent possible bias from the observer. (Parents may be in denial of their child's diagnosis with a disorder.)

2. *Key:*   Listening Skills: All are symptoms of CAPD except item number 5 (ADHD or may be TFM). Item numbers 3, 7, 8, 9, and 11 may be associated with *both* disorders.
   Academic Skills: All may be associated with *both* disorders except ADHD (item numbers 2, 5, 6, 7, and 11) and CAPD (item numbers 9, 10, and 12).
   Additional: All are symptoms of CAPD except item numbers 3, 4, 6, and 7 (ADHD) and item numbers 5 and 8 (BOTH).

APPENDIX B: VISUAL-RHYMING THERAPY*

Visual-rhyming therapy involves the integration of visual and auditory information. The clinician shows the child a list of the consonant graphemes (see below) and a target word written on an index card. The child is told to state all possible words that rhyme with the target word, beginning with the first grapheme and continuing to the final one on the chart. The target word may be *cat,* to which the child will appropriately respond, *bat, fat, hat, cat, mat, gnat, pat, rat, sat, tat, vat.* After each correct response, the child should be given a magnetic chip or a penny for positive reinforcement.

b   d   f   g   h   j   k   l   m   n

p   q   r   s   t   v   w   x   y   z

The visual-rhyming therapy provides an excellent method to enhance the child's phonemic awareness and grapheme knowledge of weekly spelling words. For example, a spelling word may be *sadly.* The

---

*Adapted from Jeanane M. Ferre, 1997.

clinician provides the word *sad* on an index card and instructs the child to rhyme every possible word to *sad*. Another example may be the spelling word *fracture*, in which the target word *act* may be provided on the index card.

Upon completion of this task, the spelling word *sadly* or *fracture* is introduced to the child, who must now correctly spell the designated spelling word on a chalkboard or a "Magna Doodle." Usually, the child has no difficulty in correctly spelling the portion of the word that has been rhymed in the visual-rhyming exercise. If the child exhibits difficulty in spelling the word, then he or she should be shown the component words that were used in therapy, and instructed to rewrite the word several times.

Initially, individuals with decoding or integration CAPD will struggle with this therapy. The child consistently will look to the clinician for a signal indicating if indeed a correct or incorrect response was provided. The child may not realize that the word *mad* rhymes with *sad* or that *gad* is not an official English word. After a few weeks of exposure to this form of therapy, the child no longer looks to the clinician for approval of his or her responses and the child's response time improves.

The goal of this therapy is to integrate visual and auditory information. As the child becomes successful at rhyming and spelling, a different visual chart may then be shown to the child (see below). This new chart includes consonant blends. The child rhymes the word on the index card to all sounds, including the consonant blends. For instance, the child properly rhymes *sad* with *bad, dad, fad, **glad**, had, lad, mad, pad, **plaid**, sad, tad.* The child may become confused when concentrating on the consonant blends and may switch the vowel sounds, such as *bad, dad, fad, **glid, hid, lid**.* To overcome this, the child may be told to give the word on the index card and then the new rhyme word, such as *sad–bad, sad–dad, sad–fad, sad–glad, sad–had, sad–lad, sad–mad.*

b	d	f	g	h	j	k	l	m
bl	dr	fl	gl			kl		
br		fr	gr			kr		

n	p	q	r	s	t	v	w	y	z
	pl			sl					
	pr			sk					

The visual-rhyming therapy compliments other forms of therapy, such as phonemic synthesis training and/or auditory discrimination in depth. Exposure to these therapeutic measures increases the child's phonemic awareness, while the utilization of the visual-rhyming therapy increases the integration of visual and auditory modalities. The children usually indicate their pleasure not only in increasing their reading and spelling skills but also in properly hearing the individual sounds.

REFERENCES

Barkley, R. A. (1990). *Attention deficit hyperactivity disorder: A handbook for diagnosis and treatment.* New York: Guilford.

Cook, J. R., Mausbach, T., Burd, L., Generoso, G., Gascon, G., Slotnick, H., Patterson, B., Johnson, R. D., Hankey, B., & Reynolds, B. (1993). A preliminary study of the relationship between central auditory processing and attention deficit disorder. *Journal of Psychiatry Neuroscience, 18*(3), 130–137.

Ferre, J. M. (1997). *Processing power: A guide to CAPD assessment and management.* San Antonio: Communication Skill Builders/The Psychological Corporation.

Gascon, G., Johnson, R., & Burd, L. (1986). Central auditory processing and attention deficit disorders. *Journal of Child Neurology, 1,* 27–33.

Ivey, R. G., & Jerome, L. (1988). *Relationship between central audition and attention deficit disorder.* Paper presented at the American Speech-Language and Hearing Association, Boston.

Katz, J. (1992). Classification of auditory processing disorders. In J. Katz, N. Stecker, & D. Henderson (Eds.), *Central auditory processing: A transdisciplinary view* (pp. 81–93). St. Louis: Mosby Year Book.

Katz, J., & Fletcher, C. (1982). *Phonemic synthesis training program.* Vancouver, WA: Precision Acoustics.

Keith, R. W. (1994). *ACPT: Auditory Continuous Performance Test, examiner's manual.* San Antonio: Harcourt Brace.

Keith, R. W., & Engineer, P. (1991). Effects of methylphenidate on the auditory processing abilities of children with ADHD. *Journal of Learning Disabilities,* 630–636.

Keller, W. (1992). Auditory processing disorder or attention deficit disorder? In J. Katz, N. Stecker, & D. Henderson (Eds.), *Central auditory processing: A transdisciplinary view* (pp. 107–114). St. Louis: Mosby Year Book.

Lindamood, C., & Lindamood, P. (1969). *Auditory discrimination in depth.* Chicago: Riverside Publications.

Tillery, K. L. (1992). *Central auditory processing abilities of attention deficit hyperactivity disordered children: With and without methylphenidate.* Unpublished master's thesis, Illinois State University.

12

MANAGEMENT OF ADOLESCENTS AND ADULTS WITH CENTRAL AUDITORY PROCESSING DISORDERS

JANE A. BARAN
University of Massachusetts, Amherst

The area of central auditory assessment has received considerable attention in both the research and clinical arenas over the past three decades. Only recently, however, has much attention been directed toward the management of individuals with central auditory processing disorders. This situation has been reflected in a common criticism that has frequently been directed at audiologists in the not-so-distant past (i.e., that audiologists were quite good at diagnosing central auditory processing disorders, but that few were adept at recommending what to do with these individuals once their disorders had been identified). Teachers, speech-language pathologists, and other professionals charged with providing services to these individuals were often frustrated by the lack of specific recommendations for meaningful therapeutic, educational, and/or support services offered for many of these individuals. Fortunately, this situation is beginning to change as evidenced by the extensive coverage of management issues addressed in this book.

Although there has been considerable interest in the development of management programs in the recent past, a perusal of the information presented in this book reveals an emphasis on management options and approaches for use with young children who present with auditory processing disorders. Relatively little attention has been directed toward management options and approaches for adults. This is due in large part to the increasing number of children with language and learning disabilities and/or attentional deficits who are being referred for central auditory assessment and for whom identification of a central auditory processing disorder necessitates the generation of a management plan. The focus on management options for use with children is also likely to be related to the fact that many of the children who we have diagnosed in the past 10 to 15 years with central auditory processing disorders have only recently matured into adolescents and adults. In spite of the fact that they have "grown" into adults, they have not "outgrown" their central auditory processing deficits. Hence, the need for management options directed at the older student is just beginning to be realized.

Finally, due to an increased awareness of central auditory processing disorders on the part of parents, teachers, and other professionals, we are beginning to see more older students being referred for the first time for assessment and management of central auditory processing disorders. Although in most of these individuals, the disorders are likely to be developmental in nature, it is only now that they are being diagnosed, as the public has become more aware of the existence of central auditory processing disorders and their potential effects on learning and academic success. For all these reasons and the pressures associated with them, attention is now being directed toward the development of intervention programs for older individuals.

As was the case with children, management approaches that are being advocated for use with adolescents and adults with central auditory processing disorders fall into three major categories. These include approaches designed to (1) improve signal quality, (2) improve auditory perceptual skills, and (3) enhance language and cognitive resources of the individual (ASHA, 1996). Although many of the specific management options used with children can and have been used with adolescents and adults, these older individuals often present unique challenges and special needs. Academic, vocational, and psychological or emotional issues often surface and/or become more severe as the individual with central auditory processing disorders matures and as processing demands increase. Additional management options—such as academic or vocational modifications, psychological counseling, career counseling, and transition programming—may be needed. Hence, there are a number of additional issues and considerations that need to be addressed when planning a management program for older individuals.

DEVELOPING A MANAGEMENT PROGRAM FOR ADOLESCENTS AND ADULTS WITH CENTRAL AUDITORY PROCESSING DISORDERS

Neural Plasticity and Age

Although it has been known for some time that the young brain is plastic and may react positively to stimulation, the evidence for the older brain is not nearly as impressive (See Chapter 2 of this book for a discussion of this issue.) Therefore, the age of the individual may influence the management options one would select. It is unlikely that significant changes or reorganization in the neural forms and connections that underlie learning and changes in behavior will occur with the older patient. Thus, management options selected for use with the older individual are likely to focus on signal enhancement options, strategy instruction, and academic and vocational modifications, with relatively less reliance on direct intervention procedures such as auditory training and speech and language intervention.

Ecological and Lifespan Perspective

Researchers are now beginning to amass data that suggest that developmental central auditory processing disorders may persist throughout an individual's life and that these disorders are frequently quite pervasive. It is now obvious, then, that a lifespan approach to management is needed for most individuals (Baran, 1996; Kleinman & Bashir, 1996). In other words, since most children diagnosed with central auditory processing disorders will not outgrow these disorders, but rather will mature into adolescents and adults with central auditory processing disorders, management programs need to be expanded to address the unique difficulties encountered by older individuals with central auditory processing disorders. Although many young children have been successfully managed with direct intervention programs and efforts toward strategy instruction in the primary and elementary school years, problems often reemerge as the child enters adolescence and adulthood, as the demands on auditory processing typically increase and the contexts in which the individual may need to function change.

The older individual is expected to function in many more contexts (family, social, job, etc.) than the child, who is typically viewed primarily in the context of school (i.e., as a learner). For the adult, the demands and skills required to function in these situations may change from situation to situation and from time to time. Even the adult who continues to find himself or herself in the context of a "learner" may find new and unique challenges to overcome. Class sizes are likely to be larger than what the individual was accustomed to as a child, for example. With the increase in class size, there may also be an increase in the background noise level of the larger classroom, and it is less likely that the instructor will be able to monitor understanding (or lack thereof) of class materials in the faces of his or her students. It is therefore essential that one use an ecological and life span perspective in planning management programs for these older individuals with central auditory processing disorders.

Comorbidity of Other Disabilities

Although auditory processing disorders may exist by themselves, it is much more frequently the case that these disorders coexist with other disorders. Common comorbid conditions include speech and language disorders, learning disabilities, attention deficit disorders with or without hyperactivity, psychological and emotional disorders, social and behavioral problems, and, in some cases, frank neurological involvement. Although there have been many attempts to establish cause-and-effect relationships between several of these disorders, the relationships remain elusive and, more than likely, not unidirectional. More critical to the successful management of the individuals with comorbid disorders than the identification of cause-and-effect relationships is the identification of the various disorders and/or disabilities that coexist so that an effective management plan can be developed that will address all areas of weakness, disabilities, and needs. Management strategies may cut across several different professional boundaries, and it is critical that professionals from a variety of disciplines provide input into the development of a management program where several comorbid conditions exist.

Interdisciplinary Approach to Assessment and Management

Because of the comorbidity of central auditory processing disorders with several other disorders, an interdisciplinary approach to both assessment and management is strongly advocated. In order to develop a clear and comprehensive understanding of the difficulties that a given individual with a central auditory processing disorder and possibly other related problems may experience, it is essential that several professionals consult to determine assessment needs and management procedures for the individual with such disabilities. One only needs to consider the variety and scope of presenting problems (see Table 12.1) to recognize the importance of such a comprehensive approach to the assessment and management of the individual with central auditory and related disabilities.

TABLE 12.1   Common Presenting Symptomatology Associated with Central Auditory Processing Disorders and Related Language and Cognitive Disorders

- Inordinate difficulty hearing in noisy or reverberant environments
- Lack of music appreciation
- Difficulty following conversations on the telephone
- Difficulty following instructions
- Difficulty taking notes
- Difficulty following long conversations
- Auditory memory deficits
- Difficulty learning a foreign language or other technical courses where the language is largely unfamiliar or novel
- Spelling difficulties
- Reading problems
- Writing problems
- Organizational problems
- Difficulty in directing, sustaining, or dividing attention
- Behavioral, psychological, and/or social problems
- Academic difficulties

Need for Education

There continues to persist a belief on the part of many individuals (e.g., faculty, administrators, employers, etc.) that most of the learning, perceptual, and behavioral difficulties one sees in young children are developmental in nature and that these individuals will simply outgrow these problems as they mature. This has been true for difficulties associated with learning disability, language-learning disabilities, attention deficit disorders, and, at least by association, central auditory processing disorders (Baran, 1996; Kleinman & Bashir, 1996; Murphy, 1996). However, one only has to look at the number of students in postsecondary programs who present with these same types of problems to recognize that these problems are not unique to childhood, but rather are life-long issues.

Unfortunately, many people with whom the individual may come into contact as he or she moves out of elementary educational programs, through secondary and/or postsecondary programs to vocational/professional placements, will not be sensitive to these issues. There remain faculty and administrators in institutions of higher education who continue to question the existence of several of these types of disabilities, and if they do acknowledge the existence of the disabilities, they do not believe that the deficits are severe enough to affect performance negatively. One continues to hear of reports where faculty and/or administrators refuse to accept a previous diagnosis of learning disability or central auditory processing disorders and require that the diagnosis be current. A recent example of this that has received widespread press coverage was the decision of a Boston University President-Designate who decided that students would be required to provide documentation of their learning problems obtained within the past three years to continue to be eligible for academic accommodations and support services (Lewin, 1996).

In other instances, faculty members have refused to offer accommodations recommended by appropriately certified and licensed professionals who have deemed that certain accommodations are reasonable and appropriate. In some cases, faculty members have been reported to be conducting their own "learning disabilities assessment" by asking the student to read, write, or perform some other academic task. Such faculty then make a decision based on *their* assessment, and not one offered by the professionals with expertise in the area of disability—whether the individual has a language, learning, or auditory processing disorder.

To this day, there are speech-language pathologists who claim that none of their clients has auditory processing disorders, yet these clinicians have huge caseloads of children and adults diagnosed with language-learning disabilities, specific language impairment, and other related disorders. Obviously, the need for education is great. If we are to adequately serve the needs of adolescents and adults with central auditory processing disorders, we are going to need to enlist the cooperation of all of these individuals. Much of the intervention may involve procedures that we cannot provide without the assistance of professionals from outside our discipline (e.g., modifications of course requirements, provision of alternative tests, changes in teaching styles, etc.).

INTERVENTION/MANAGEMENT OPTIONS

Many of the intervention and management options available for use with the older client have been discussed in detail elsewhere in this book. Therefore, comments on areas that have received considerable coverage in other chapters will be limited, for the most part, to discussions of modifications of these procedures for use with the older patient. The reader is cautioned that different terms may be used in this chapter than in other chapters. This potential difference in the use of terminology reflects the lack of consistency in the use of terminology to describe procedures in the literature dealing with intervention programs. Therefore, if a procedure discussed here appears to resemble a procedure that carries a different title in another chapter, it is likely that both chapters are addressing the same underlying procedure.

Auditory Training

Several of the chapters in this book have addressed the issue of auditory training. These types of intervention have proved to be useful, particularly with the young child. Auditory training programs focusing on development temporal processing skills such as those developed by Tallal and Merzenich and their colleagues have begun to be subjected to empirical testing and are being shown to be effective with young children (Merzenich et al., 1996; Tallal et al., 1996). There is, however, limited information on the efficacy of such direct auditory training programs with adults. Given this lack of efficacy data and the comments earlier regarding brain plasticity in adults (i.e., the decreased likelihood of significant changes in the neural forms and connections underlying auditory processing skills and abilities as one matures into adulthood), application of direct intervention programs are likely to enjoy only limited application with the older individual with central processing disorders at this time. The reader who is interested in a discussion of the specific auditory training procedures that have been used with patients with central auditory processing disorders is referred to in Parts II and III of this book.

Signal Enhancement

Chapter 6 of this book provides an excellent review of the application of FM technology in the management of the individual with a central auditory processing disorder. Personal FM systems can be used to increase significantly the signal-to-noise ratio of a speaker's voice in the presence of a competing noise source, and thus increase the likelihood that an individual will be able to process auditory information in a more efficient manner. Such technology should be given serious consideration as a viable option for an individual with a variety of auditory problems (e.g., problems hearing in noisy or reverberant environments, difficulty with following lectures in large classroom environments, difficulty with directing and/or maintaining auditory attention, etc.). A potential limiting factor, however, is the age of the individual when one first attempts to fit a personal FM system. Experience has indicated that if a personal FM system is not dispensed at an early age, prognosis for successful introduction of the technology in the adolescence years is limited. This is partly due to the need on the part of adolescents to be perceived as part of the group and not be perceived as different.

I am unaware of large-scale efforts to utilize personal FM systems with older individuals. However, prognosis for success is likely to be good if one can get around issues of rejection of the instrumentation for self-esteem and peer acceptance reasons. An alternative to the personal FM system that may provide assistance and is not nearly as dependent on personal acceptance issues is the use of classroom amplification systems (Ray, Sarff, & Glassford, 1984). An additional benefit of the use of such a system is that all individuals within the amplified environment can benefit from the enhanced signal-to-noise ratio.

Other procedures designed to specifically improve signal quality should also be entertained. These would include acoustic modifications of the classroom or listening environment, provision of telephone amplifying devices to aid understanding of employees who work around sources of noise that would interfere with understanding of the speaker's message, application of FM technology for purposes of tape-recording class lectures, and others.

Language and Cognitive Interventions

As was the case for interventions directed at development of auditory perceptual skills, speech and language and/or cognitive intervention procedures used with the older individual are less likely to focus on specific skill acquisition (e.g., phonological awareness or decoding, development of syntactic skills, etc.) and more likely to focus on development of metalinguistic and metacognitive skills and strategy development. Since specific deficit areas are not likely to be remediated in most older individuals with developmental language and/or cognitive disabilities, management efforts are more likely to be directed at teaching students how to compensate for their deficits so that they will not interfere with overall academic and social performance. For instance, to reduce the likelihood that poor phonological processing skills will result in significant reading comprehension problems, students may be taught how to derive meaning from context rather than how to decode individual words. Of particular significance here is the discussion of strategy instruction that follows. Chapters 4, 5, and 8 provide information on several language and cognitive interventions that have been utilized successfully with children with auditory processing and related disorders. Additional information specific to management of adults with language-learning disabilities can be found in Kleinman and Bashir (1996).

STRATEGY INSTRUCTION

A number of strategies have been used with individuals with central auditory processing disorders and related learning disorders. Although many of the strategies suggested appear to be obvious and therefore would appear to require little introduction other than identification or specification of the strategy, this may not be the case for the individual with the disability. If these strategies were so readily apparent, it is likely that the individual would be using the strategy or strategies on his or her own. Therefore, many professionals are advocating for formalized strategy instruction procedures. Several models have been proposed, with most of these being recommended for group instruction. Although designed for use with groups of students, many can be modified for individual use.

One such model proposed by Deschler and associates (Deschler, Alley, Warner, & Schumaker, 1981; Deschler, Schumaker, Lenz, & Ellis, 1984) involves eight steps (see Figure 12.1). The first step involves the pretesting of strategy usage to determine if the student is applying the strategy. This typically would be followed by a discussion of the value of the strategy use and a commitment on the part of the student to master the strategy. The second step targets a description of the new strategy and focuses on the identification of the elements of the strategy and the methods of appli-

FIGURE 12.1 Recommended Steps in the Application of Learning-Strategies Instruction as Advocated by Deschler and Associates

Step 1: Pretest and Commitment

Step 2: Description of the Strategies

Step 3: Modeling the Strategies

Step 4: Verbal Rehearsal of Strategies

Step 5: Controlled Practice and Feedback

Step 6: Grade/Age-Appropriate Practice and Feedback

Step 7: Posttest & Communication to Generalization

Step 8: Generalization

Source: Deschler's steps adapted from William M. Bender, *Learning Disabilities: Characteristics, Identification, and Teaching Strategies* (2nd ed.). Boston: Allyn and Bacon. Copyright © by Allyn and Bacon. Adapted by permission.

cation of the strategy. Alternative strategies may also be considered at this stage. Step 3 is dedicated to the modeling of the behavior or strategy for the student. The teacher or other professional initially describes each step in the strategy as each step is initiated and then several different tasks are completed to demonstrate the function of the strategy.

Step 4 involves verbal rehearsal of the strategy by the student. Each student is required to identify the action to be taken in each step of the strategy and explain why each step is important to the overall strategy. The fifth step involves practice with materials that have been controlled for level of difficulty so as not to hinder mastery of the strategy. This is followed by application of the strategy to grade appropriate materials in the next step. Performance is typically charted to show changes in performance over time as the strategy is applied. The last steps involve generalization and postinstruction testing. The student is trained to apply the strategy to new materials from the mainstream class and strategy usage is periodically reassessed.

A similar program has been developed by Harris, Graham, and Pressley (1991). In this approach, the student is expected to progress through seven stages (see Figure 12.2). During Stage 1 *(preskill development)*, preskills required for the understanding, acquisition, and execution of the targeted strategy that are not already in the learner's skill base are developed. Stage 2 *(review of current performance level)* involves the instructor and the learner examining and discussing any baseline data available and any strategies that the individual currently uses. During this phase of instruction, negative or ineffective strategies or self-statements may be discussed and the potential benefits of the proposed strategy are highlighted. Finally, a commitment to participation as a partner in the instruction is required and goals are established in a collaborative manner.

In Stage 3 *(discuss the executive strategy)*, the executive strategy is described in detail by the instructor, who also provides the learner with indications for strategy use and the potential benefits that may be derived from use of the strategy. During Stage 4 *(model the strategy and self-instructions)*, the instructor or a peer models the strategy to be learned and the effectiveness of the model's performance is discussed. The student is expected to generate his or her own self-instructions to direct the use of the strategy, and the student and instructor may collaborate on any changes that may make the strategy more effective. In Stage 5 *(mastery of the strategy)*, the student is expected to memorize the steps in the strategy and the self-instructions and to describe the steps and self-instructions to the instructor. Students are permitted to paraphrase the specific requirements for each step in the strategy application as long as the meaning remains intact.

FIGURE 12.2   Basic Stages in Self-Regulated Strategy Development Proposed by Harris, Graham, and Pressley (1991)

Step 1: Develop preskills.

Step 2: Review currently used strategies.

Step 3: Discuss the executive strategy.

Step 4: Model the strategy.

Step 5: Memorize the strategy.

Step 6: Practice the strategy.

Step 7: Use the strategy independently.

Source: Adapted from Harris, Graham, & Pressley, 1991.

Stage 6 *(collaborative practice of strategy steps and self-instructions)* activities center on student practice of the strategy and supporting self-instructional activities while performing the tasks. Additionally, self-regulation procedures such as goal setting, self-monitoring, and self-reinforcement are discussed, mutually agreed upon by student and instructor, and implemented by the student throughout this phase of training. Prompts, interventions, and suggestions offered by the instructor to facilitate strategy use are gradually faded over practice sessions until the student achieves independent performance on the use of the strategy. As the student gains competence, more challenging goals are determined cooperatively, and criterion levels are gradually increased until the final goal is met and plans are made for the transfer and maintenance of the strategy.

During the final stage, Stage 7 *(independent performance)*, transition to covert self-instruction is encouraged as the student learns to use the strategy independently. Self-regulation procedures are continued in this stage and plans for transfer and maintenance of the strategy are undertaken. One additional feature of the program is that instruction through-out the program is criterion based and the stages are considered to be flexible and recursive, allowing for individualized programming to meet different students' needs.

Academic/Vocational Modifications

It is not uncommon for individuals with central auditory processing dis-orders and other related cognitive, language, and learning problems to experience difficulties both in academic and vocational placements. Pro-fessionals have for years had experience in working with children with language and learning disabilities in the primary grades, and to some degree, the secondary grades. Only recently, however, have professionals been called on to assist in providing recommendations for academic modifications for adult students. This is due in large part to the fact that until the enactment of recent federal and/or state mandates, most stu-dents with significant learning problems did not gain admission to insti-tutions of higher education. Admission requirements, most notability the Scholastic Aptitude Test (SAT) requirement, often prevented many stu-dents from meeting admission requirements. With federal and/or state mandates now in place that require admission requirements to be mod-ified for students with documented disabilities, many more students are in college classrooms.

Secondary and postsecondary programs present unique challenges to students with disabilities. Classes are frequently larger, particularly in postsecondary programs, where freshmen typically are enrolled in courses designed to meet the general education or core requirements specified by their college or university. Faculty are less likely to get to know each student individually and carefully monitor each individual's progress and areas of need, and there is a greater reliance on indepen-dent learning on the part of the student. All of these factors can lead to new and/or increased difficulties for the student with learning problems.

Recognizing the need for individualized academic planning, many colleges and universities have begun to develop academic support ser-vices for their students with learning disabilities. Researchers are there-fore beginning to amass some data regarding the unique problems of the older student and the challenges that universities face in attempting to meet the special needs of this population. However, the range of services available from one institution to another is quite broad, and even in those institutions with the more extensive programs, services available to students are not likely to match the types available to them in their elementary and secondary school placements.

Equally as important are the vocational modifications that may be needed when one leaves an academic program (either secondary, post-secondary, or technical training) and enters the vocational workplace. In this area, there is little in the way of services available for individuals with special needs. At the present time, assistance is typically provided only through consultation with the employer, and little data are available to support the efficacy or any modifications of accommodations that may be recommended.

Table 12.2 provides a listing of some common academic modifications that can be used to assist adult learners. Some of these modifications are more realistic for secondary students, whereas others have greater application with post-secondary students. For example, seating is typically not assigned by the instructor in college courses. In these cases, although preferential seating may be desirable, it would typically be the student's responsibility to secure such preferential seating. On the other hand, in college courses, it is common practice for faculty to provide students with a syllabus at the beginning of the semester that outlines course objectives, course requirements, materials to be covered in the class, and the sequence of material coverage, as well as reading assignments. It is therefore unlikely that a student would require that reading assignments be provided ahead of class instruction. However, the same is not necessarily true for high school courses.

TABLE 12.2 Examples of Academic Modifications for Students in Secondary and Postsecondary Academic Placements

- Untimed tests
- Alternative test formats
- Test administration in alternative environments (e.g., less noisy, less distractions)
- Provision of notetaking services
- Provision of tutoring services (may also include peer tutoring)
- Reduced courseloads
- Creative scheduling of classes to ensure that course requirements and task demands are equally distributed over the course of the academic program
- Substitution or waiver of academic requirements (e.g., foreign language)
- Preferential seating (if seating is assigned)
- Tape recording of lectures and presentations
- Video recording of lectures and presentations
- Assignment or selection of course section where instructor's teaching philosophy and style are consistent with student needs
- Provision of outlines, lecture notes, or reading assignments prior to class presentation so that students can review materials in advance

A major concern for many students with central auditory processing disorders and related disorders is the ability to meet a foreign language requirement. Some universities will waive students from the requirement if a disability is documented. Many more, however, will not waive the requirement, but will insist that the requirement be modified. Most commonly, the modification of a foreign language requirement is the substitution of a "culture" course. A second accommodation that some universities have allowed is the substitution of a course on American Sign Language. Obviously, this particular accommodation would be especially helpful for the individual with a significant auditory processing disorder, since the reliance on auditory skills for acquisition of the language is significantly reduced.

Career Counseling and Transition Programming

A major need of the older individual with central auditory processing disorder is in the area of career counseling and transition planning. Many adolescents and young adults do not fully appreciate how their learning or communication problems may interact with job demands to set them up for frustration, possible failure, and loss of self-esteem. Often, students may be guided through the use of appropriate counseling techniques to more appropriate career choices if they can identify their strengths and weaknesses and explore the variety of career options that are open to them. Frequently, parental or societal pressures push students into career choices for which they are ill equipped, uninterested, and unmotivated. Counseling may help the student learn how to deal with these parental and/or societal pressures and how to become more self-assertive.

Even when a good match is found between an individual's interests, skills, and career or educational choices, it is likely that the individual with a disability will encounter new problems as he or she moves from one context to another (e.g., from school to employment). Exploration of the potential difficulties that may be encountered in the new context prior to the time that they are actually encountered may help the individual plan how he or she will react to these difficulties. Finally, an essential component of transition planning for the individual with an auditory processing or related disorder is self-advocacy training.

Self-Advocacy Training

As alluded to earlier, as the individual matures from childhood into adolescence and into adulthood, the likelihood that he or she will have a case manager, advocate, or other professional to advocate for his or her needs becomes increasing smaller. Young students often become dependent on these individuals and do not develop the skills and abilities needed to take on this role (i.e., advocacy) themselves as the need arises. As a consequence, they may struggle in new and difficult situations rather than ask for assistance and/or reasonable accommodations. This is particularly true at the postsecondary level, where many students feel that faculty are unapproachable, or, in some cases, that a faculty will be biased against them if they disclose their disabilities or deficits when they ask for assistance or accommodations.

Although such problems related to poor development of self-advocacy skills are often noted in postsecondary environments, they also occur in vocational settings and may be equally as problematic for the employee. An employee who is not able to advocate for one's needs may find that he or she is at risk for job loss or employment termination because of perceived employee ineffectiveness. The individual may also find that he or she is being passed over for promotions or that he or she is not accepted by colleagues in the workplace because of being perceived as aloof or antisocial.

MANAGEMENT OF PATIENTS WITH COMPROMISE OF THE PERIPHERAL AND CENTRAL AUDITORY SYSTEMS

The previous section of this chapter focused on the management of central auditory processing disorders in individuals with normal peripheral hearing sensitivity. Central auditory processing disorders, however, may coexist with, or be secondary to, peripheral hearing loss in many individuals. In these cases, determination of the presence of a central auditory processing impairment is critical to the successful management of the patient with a hearing loss. Unfortunately, current practice patterns tend to focus on assessment of the function of the auditory periphery and subsequent hearing aid selection and fitting procedures. Assessment of the integrity and function of the central auditory nervous system of patients receive little, if any, attention.

Today, most individuals with hearing loss are considered to be viable candidates for amplification, given the advances that have occurred in hearing aid technology over the past several years. In addition, since the benefits of binaural amplification have been clearly established in the literature, binaural fittings have become the standard of care, even in cases where asymmetrical hearing losses have been identified. In spite of the obvious benefits of binaural fittings for the majority of patients, there exists a subgroup of patients with hearing loss for whom binaural fittings may be contraindicated. In addition, there exists a second group of patients for whom amplification may not be contraindicated but whose success with amplification is limited by the presence of a central auditory processing disorder. In these cases, identification of the presence of a central auditory processing disorder, which may be the limiting factor, should allow the audiologist to set realistic expectations for the hearing aid user and ultimately result in a more satisfied consumer.

Several investigators have reported on cases where the presentation of auditory information to the two ears of a individual with a hearing loss has resulted in poorer performance than when the same information was presented to only one ear. This phenomena has been referred to in the literature as *binaural interference* and has obvious implications for the management of the patient with hearing loss. In one representative study, Jerger, Silman, Lew, and Chmiel (1993) provided evidence of binaural interference in four patients. Aided binaural speech recognition scores were derived for three of their four patients under three test conditions: monaural right ear fitting, monaural left ear fitting, and binaural fitting. In all three cases, clearly asymmetrical performance was evident for aided speech recognition measures during monaural assessments in spite of symmetrical pure tone findings. More interesting, however, was the finding that the binaural fitting resulted in a significantly poorer score when compared with the aided speech recognition score of the better ear in each of these individuals.

These investigators also provided electrophysiologic evidence of binaural interference for three patients. Middle latency responses were derived with monaural right, monaural left, and binaural stimulation procedures. In each of the three patients, the NaPa wave complex derived from one of the ears was noticeably larger and more normally distributed over the scalp than was the response derived from the second ear. As was the case with the speech recognition scores, however, the responses derived with binaural stimulation were markedly poorer than the responses derived from the better ear in each of the three individuals. In these types of situations (i.e., asymmetrical auditory findings), the normal expectation would be that binaural presentation of auditory information should result in either an enhancement of binaural performance over monaural performance, or a binaural performance that at least equals that of the better monaural test performance.

In these four patients, it appears that presentation of auditory information to the second or poorer ear interfered in some manner with the processing of information presented to the better ear. Although the mechanisms underlying such a phenomenon are not understood, it is likely that some type of distortion is introduced by the peripheral or central auditory system. An obvious implication of these findings is that binaural processes must work appropriately if a client with a hearing aid is to make optimum use of binaural amplification. Additional discussion of the potential influence of binaural interference and other central auditory processing mechanisms on successful management of the client with a hearing aid can be found in Musiek and Baran (1996).

Given the foregoing comments and observations, the inclusion of central auditory assessment in patients with peripheral hearing impairment should be given serious consideration. Although central auditory assessment would appear to be desirable for all hearing aid candidates, financial constraints are likely to limit this extensive application of central auditory test batteries. Diagnostic central auditory assessments are not likely to become the standard of care for all patients being considered for amplification (at least not in the foreseeable future). Thus, Musiek and Baran (1996) have suggested three different scenarios or approaches that could be used to ensure that status of the central auditory nervous system is given some attention (see Figure 12.3).

In the first scenario, patients with histories of neurologic involvement would be administered a central auditory screening test in conjunction with the audiologic evaluation or subsequent to it, but in all cases prior to hearing aid fitting. In this way, patients who are considered to be at risk for compromise of the central auditory nervous system would be given a screening test to determine the need for further diagnostic testing.

In the second scenario, all patients considered to be candidates for hearing aid fittings would be given a screening test for central function prior to the fitting of the hearing aid. Although not specifically mentioned in Musiek and Baran's discussion of these scenarios, the obvious implication of a failure on the screening test would be the need for additional diagnostic testing prior to initiation of hearing aid selection and fitting procedures for those individuals who failed the initial screening test.

In the final scenario, patients would undergo customary audiologic testing as well as hearing aid selection and fitting procedures. Only those patients who return reporting unsatisfactory performance or benefits, or those patients who do not appear to be deriving the anticipated benefits (i.e., the audiologist's expectations) from their hearing aid(s) based on follow-up procedures would be seen for central auditory testing. This testing would be completed following initial fitting procedures, but prior to the expiration of the patient's trial period so that changes in the fitting can be made without financial costs or losses to the patient.

A number of issues need to be given consideration when selecting central auditory tests for use with patients with peripheral hearing loss and when attempting to select a central test to be used as a screening instrument. The audiologist interested in the application of central auditory processing assessment with patients with peripheral hearing losses will need to carefully select those central tests that are not likely to be affected to any significant degree by the presence of a peripheral hearing impairment. In addition, the selection of a screening instrument may

FIGURE 12.3   Three Scenarios Demonstrating How Central Auditory Testing Could Be Integrated in a Management Plan for Individuals with Peripheral Hearing Impairments

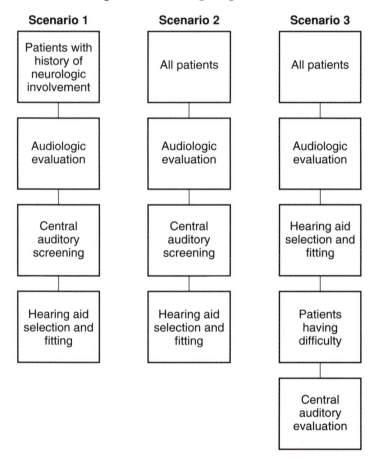

Scenario 1	Scenario 2	Scenario 3
Patients with history of neurologic involvement	All patients	All patients
Audiologic evaluation	Audiologic evaluation	Audiologic evaluation
Central auditory screening	Central auditory screening	Hearing aid selection and fitting
Hearing aid selection and fitting	Hearing aid selection and fitting	Patients having difficulty
		Central auditory evaluation

Source: Adapted from F. E. Musiek & J. A. Baran, Central auditory processing disorders in children and adults, in M. Valente (Ed.), *Hearing aids: Standards, options, and limitations* (New York: Thieme Medical Publishers, 1996). Used by permission.

not be as straightforward as it might appear because of the complexity of the structure and function of the central auditory nervous system. A comprehensive discussion of these issues is beyond the scope of this chapter. The reader interested in these topics is referred to Musiek and Baran (1996) and to Musiek, Baran, and Pinheiro (1994) for further discussion.

This section of the chapter discussed management issues surrounding the initial selection and fitting of hearing aids to patients with hearing losses. These patients are also likely to need and benefit from several of the other management issues discussed earlier. Obviously, communication enhancement training (i.e., speech-reading training) would be indicated for most, if not all, of these individuals. Other management options discussed in the preceding sections of this chapter may be indicated, depending on the specific needs of the individual.

CONCLUSION

The communication and learning difficulties encountered by an adolescent or an adult with a central auditory processing disorder often are complex, are context sensitive, and fall within the practice domains of several different professionals. It is therefore critical that management plans be formulated using both an ecological as well as an interdisciplinary perspective. Individual differences in learning and personality styles, together with the cognitive and perceptual strengths and weaknesses that the individual brings to the management program, will affect the success that one can expect with each of the management options discussed in this and other chapters. Therefore, comprehensive assessment of the individual's academic strengths and weaknesses, learning and cognitive styles, speech and language functioning, social and emotional functioning, and other related behaviors and functions should be undertaken whenever indicated.

Consideration of presenting information by professionals from the various disciplines that would typically be involved in the assessment of the behaviors outlined here should lead to realistic and cost-effective recommendations for test-needed assessments. Moreover, consultation with professionals in related fields is essential to the successful management of the individual with auditory processing disorders and other learning disabilities and disorders. Whenever feasible, an *interdisciplinary team approach* to assessment and management of these individuals is considered desirable. If the construction of such a team is not feasible for financial or logistical reasons, then a *transdisciplinary approach* encompassing consultations among the professionals involved in the assessment of the individual is advocated.

Finally, since it appears that most developmental central auditory processing disorders persist into adolescence and beyond, a life-long approach to management is indicated. Management strategies and approaches that provided assistance to the young child may not prove to be efficient and useful for the adult. Therefore, management plans need to be periodically reevaluated and reconfigured to meet the ever-changing needs of the individual as he or she matures.

REFERENCES

American Speech-Language-Hearing Association. (1996). Central auditory processing current status of research and implications for practice. Task force on central auditory processing consensus development. *American Journal of Audiology, 5*(2), 41–54.

Baran, J. A. (1996). Audiologic evaluation and management of adults with auditory processing disorders. *Seminars in Speech and Language, 17,* 233–244.

Deschler, D. D., Alley, G. R., Warner, M. M., & Schumaker, J. B. (1981). Instructional practices for promoting skill acquisition and generalization in severely learning disabled adolescents. *Learning Disability Quarterly, 4,* 415–421.

Deschler, D. D., Schumaker, J. B., Lenz, B. K., & Ellis, E. S. (1984). Academic and cognitive interactions for LD adolescents. Part II. *Journal of Learning Disabilities, 17,* 170–187.

Harris, K. R., Graham, S., & Pressley, M. (1991). Cognitive-behavioral approaches in reading and written language: Developing self-regulated learners. In N. N. Singh, & I. L. Beale (Eds.), *Learning disabilities: Nature, theory, and treatment* (pp. 415–451). New York: Springer-Verlag.

Jerger, J., Silman, S., Lew, H. L., & Chmiel, R. (1993). Case studies in binaural interference: Converging evidence from behavioral and electrophysiologic measures. *Journal of the American Academy of Audiology, 4,* 122–131.

Kleinman, S. N., & Bashir, A. S. (1996). Adults with language-learning disabilities: New challenges and changing perspectives. *Seminars in Speech and Language, 17,* 201–216.

Lewin, T. (1996). College gets tougher on verifying learning disabilities. *The New York Times,* February 13, p. A16.

Merzenich, M. M., Jenkins, W. M., Johnston, P., Schreiner, C., Miller, S. L., & Tallal, P. (1996). Temporal processing deficits of language-learning impaired children ameliorated by training. *Science, 271,* 77–81.

Murphy, K. (1996). Adults with attention deficit hyperactivity disorder: Assessment and treatment considerations. *Seminars in Speech and Language, 17,* 245–254.

Musiek, F. E., & Baran, J. A. (1996). Hearing aids and the central auditory nervous system. In M. Valente (Ed.), *Hearing aids: Standards, options, and limitations* (pp. 407–438). New York: Thieme Medical Publishers.

Musiek, F. E., Baran, J. A., & Pinheiro, M. L. (1994). *Neuroaudiology: Case studies.* San Diego: Singular Publishing Group.

Ray, H., Sarff, L. S., & Glassford, J. E. (1984). Sound field amplification: An innovative educational intervention for mainstreamed learning disabled students. *The Directive Teacher,* Summer/Fall, 18–20.

Tallal, P., Miller, S. L., Bedi, G., Byma, G., Wang, X., Nagarajan, S. S., Schreiner, C., Jenkins, W. M., & Merzenich, M. M. (1996). Language comprehension in language-learning impaired children improved with acoustically modified speech. *Science, 271,* 81–84.

13

CENTRAL AUDITORY PROCESSING AND COCHLEAR IMPLANT THERAPY

JACK KATZ
State University of New York at Buffalo

This chapter deals with a central auditory processing (CAP) approach to improve cochlear implant (CI) effectiveness in adults. The relationship between CAP and CIs may not be obvious. After all, CAP represents a problem at the level of the brain or brain stem, whereas severe to profound hearing loss generally involves the cochlea.

To better understand the relationship, let us start with a definition of CAP. For many years, we have considered CAP to be "what we do with what we hear" (Lasky & Katz, 1983). People learn to perceive auditory information crudely from earliest childhood, and, with time, they improve on their listening efficiency. Speech concepts are "hard-wired" into the brain by adulthood, explaining why even a normal adult hearer has difficulty learning a foreign dialect.

The signal sent by the cochlear implant through the auditory system is far different from the signal received by the brain in earlier years, whether the individual had normal hearing or learned to perceive through a hearing aid. There is a major discrepancy between what he or she interpreted as speech and the patterns delivered by the CI. This might be akin to hearing a person speak in a strange tongue. The sounds appear unfamiliar, imprecise, and too quick to catch.

The difference between the earlier signals, gathered and refined over the years, and the new CI signal can be illustrated by two anecdotes. One CI wearer initially thought that everyone had whistles in their throats when he heard speech through the device. The sounds were meaningless and annoying. Another person could not distinguish speech from pure-tones. In time, and with therapy, both of these users derived excellent benefits from their implants.

Because the new speech patterns provide such a strange message and because sounds never before heard are now highly audible, the listener with a CI has an engram mismatch. That is, the speech concepts encoded in the brain, as well as the decoding strategies of the past, no longer apply well to the CI signal. Except in the most fortunate postlingually deafened individuals, one can expect major confusions and listening inefficiencies. Although these difficulties tend to be resolved over time, the effort is a long one and the project often incomplete.

When one CI user was told that she would be working on the *H*-sound, she said, "But *H* doesn't have a sound; it's just air coming out." When asked to make the *H*-sound into a microphone, she was amazed how loud the sound was. When she was given the sounds /*m, e, k*/ and asked to put them together to make a word, she combined them but was unable to give the word. When told it was *make*, she was surprised "that *make* has a *K* at the end. I thought it was a silent *K*." Despite two years of successful implant use, this individual did not overcome many of the misconceptions learned during her years of deafness.

Clearly, not all of the confusions are corrected when one is given the opportunity to hear. Some of the percepts need to be trained, especially in the prelingually deaf. The NIH Consensus Statement on Adults and Children with Cochlear Implants (1995) states that training and educational intervention are necessary for optimal results. Further, prelingually deafened adults may need different types of help and require longer periods of therapy than postlingually deafened adults.

CAP CONCEPTS AND CI THERAPY

Although the CI user is likely to have had an efficient auditory processing system prior to implant, the patterns arising from the new device are so different and the range of frequencies so much broader that the brain is inefficient in dealing with these signals. The typical CI wearer improves from a severe corner audiogram to a mild loss across the entire audiometric range; however, the usefulness of this new hearing for understanding speech is more limited.

Good gains are reported in understanding with lip reading, but CI wearers typically have limited open-set word recognition (NIH Consensus Statement, 1995). Osberger (1990) suggested that a typical word recognition score for a patient with a CI is roughly 14 percent, although better scores are obtained when using the newer processors. A serious limitation is that "prelingually deafened adults show little improvement in speech perception scores"; however, they get satisfaction from hearing environmental sounds (NIH Consensus Statement, 1995, p. 9).

By all accounts, there is a need for therapeutic intervention to get optimal results from a CI. We have tried a CAP approach in therapy both because of the somewhat limited results that have been reported in the literature, and because of the similarity between imperception of CI users and CAP cases with poor phonemic decoding abilities.

CAP Categories

CAP has been divided into four major components (Katz & Smith, 1991; Katz, 1992): (1) decoding—primarily at the phonemic level, (2) tolerance-fading memory—both short-term memory and poor speech recognition in noise, (3) integration—especially auditory-visual, and (4) organization—organizing and maintaining proper sequence. The problem faced by the CI user is similar to that of the poor decoder.

Decoding problems are described as difficulty in quickly and accurately comprehending speech, especially at the phonemic level. The CI wearer, like the person listening to a foreign language, is unable to keep up with the rapidity of the new speech patterns. That is, words may only resemble the pattern of sound the person had understood before, or, in many cases, without benefit of lip reading, the components of these words may be completely incomprehensible.

CAP Therapy for Phonemic Decoding Difficulties

A therapeutic approach has been used for many years to train children who have phonemic decoding problems associated with learning disabilities (Katz & Burge, 1971; Katz & Medol, 1972). The purpose of this work has been to strengthen their knowledge of individual phonemes and to enable them to manipulate these units. This is accomplished with phonemic discrimination drills and, even more so, with phonemic synthesis training (Katz, 1983). Phonemic analysis has also been incorporated into this therapy once the previous levels have been mastered.

In each of these therapeutic procedures, individual speech sounds are presented. Many of them are not properly perceived by the child with learning disabilities until the sounds are isolated. Older children often show surprise when they learn the sound they have heard. As the child's phonemic perception improves, positive changes are seen in the decoding of words and sentences, even though little work is carried out with suprasegmentals.

Needs of the CI Recipients

Unlike the child with a learning disability associated with CAPD, the CI user has great difficulty comprehending open-set, auditory-only speech, even when spoken slowly and distinctly. The child who is learning disabled may have a vague concept of some phonemes, but the adult prelingually deaf person may have no concept at all of many of the sounds. The adult has depended on coarticulated influences on surrounding sounds, lip reading, and context to figure out what was said. His or her previous auditory strategies provide limited success because of the weak concepts that were encoded and because of the great changes in the pattern delivered to the brain.

The child with CAPD may have moderately impaired phonemic skills, but the prelingually deafened CI wearer is likely to have a profound CAPD. This may account for the minimal improvement in speech perception seen in prelingually deafened adults. Thus, in planning encoding-decoding therapy for the patient who has a CI, especially the prelingually deafened, it is important to begin by treating the problem as a profound and tenacious one.

SUBJECTS

This report involves two prelingually deafened adults who were seen for at least one year of phonemic therapy. Both of them were identified as hearing impaired by the age of 2 years. They did not develop speech and oral language on their own, but rather required intensive training. Both subjects are intelligent and highly motivated.

Patient 1

Jack, a 24-year-old male, began phonemic training six months after receiving his implant. As a child, he was fitted with a hearing aid in his right ear. He had the CI operation at age 23 because he was disabled by the dizziness that resulted from the high level of amplification. The Nucleus-22 device was implanted in the right ear. Jack uses the SPEAK coding strategy with a Spectra processor (BP+3 setting). His audiograms before and after surgery are shown in Figure 13.1.

Jack received excellent results from the implant prior to therapy. Both his understanding and his speech production improved significantly. Prior to his CI, he earned a B.A. degree in English and is now pursuing a graduate degree.

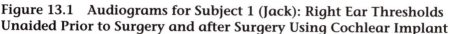

Figure 13.1   Audiograms for Subject 1 (Jack): Right Ear Thresholds Unaided Prior to Surgery and after Surgery Using Cochlear Implant

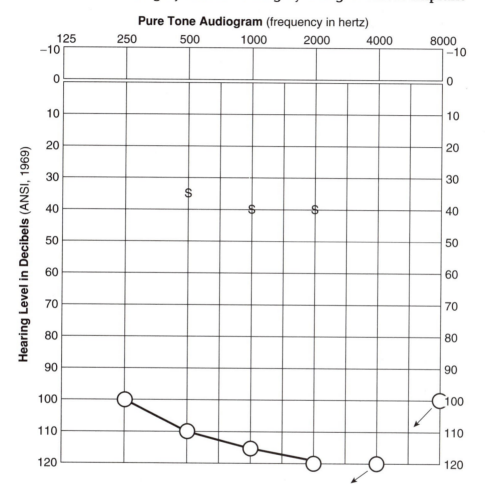

Patient 2

Carol, a 41-year-old female, began phonemic therapy 10 months after implantation. She began wearing a hearing aid in her right ear as a young child. She had the CI operation because of limited benefit from her hearing aid. The Nucleus-22 device was implanted in the left ear, even though Carol had never worn a hearing aid on that side (questionable neural survival). It was chosen because she could continue to use a hearing aid in her right ear if the surgery failed. Carol uses the SPEAK coding strategy with a Spectra processor (BP+1 setting). Her puretone audiograms before and after surgery are shown in Figure 13.2.

Carol had a fair amount of benefit from her implant prior to therapy. Her speech improved and she was able to experience environmental sounds. With the implant and lip reading, Carol was able to perform better than she had when lip reading with her hearing aid.

Despite her dyslexia, Carol went to the National Technical Institute for the Deaf and later received her bachelor's degree in special education at a private college. Presently, she works at a school for the deaf as a teacher's aide, serving children with multiple disabilities. She is considering returning to school to further her education.

Figure 13.2   Audiograms for Subject 2 (Carol): Left Ear Thresholds Unaided Prior to Surgery and after Surgery Using Cochlear Implant

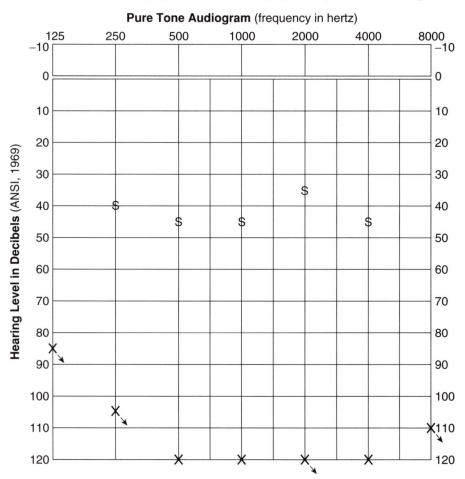

EVALUATION

Prior to and during the course of therapy, a number of auditory tests were administered to determine overall level of skill and specific phonemic confusions. Testing was carried out without benefit of visual cues. There was little concern for the visual or auditory-visual abilities of these subjects, but a great deal of concern for their hearing-only mode. Feedback to the patients on these tests was in the form of general statements or summary data. The various test lists were randomized and infrequently repeated.

Phoneme Recognition Test (PRT)

The Phoneme Recognition Test (PRT) was the primary measure used to evaluate and monitor performance. It contains 68 items, made up of two scramblings of 34 phonemes (20 consonants and 14 vowels). The PRT score was recorded in percent correct. The test was originally given recorded, but our subjects were not pleased with the recorded version, hearing sounds and distortions not obvious to the normal ear. Eventually, we heeded the sage words of Parkin and Dankowski (1986) and used live voice testing only. Although this form lacks the consistency of a recorded test, live voice is the more realistic signal and was more acceptable to the patients.

To ensure reliability in presentation of phonemes and recording patient responses, different clinicians tested and then retested patients. The results showed excellent reliability. However, initial training was necessary to ensure that each clinician produced the sounds properly and that the scoring system was clearly understood.

Word Recognition Scores (WRS)

Word recognition scores (WRS) were obtained using NU-6s for Jack and W-22s for Carol. WRS enabled us to monitor whether benefits seen in the phonemic therapy had generalized to the perception of words. These tests were scored both in the percentage of words correct and the percentage of sounds correct.

CID Every Day Sentences

Every Day Sentences test was administered to determine the patients' ability to apply their new phonemic knowledge in longer speech units. The test was scored in percentage of words correctly identified based on 50 key words from the 10 sentences.

THERAPY PROCEDURES

The therapy program was intended to (1) teach the patient what each phoneme sounded like through the CI, (2) help the person discriminate each sound from the others, (3) provide sufficient repetition to enable longer storage and better retrieval, (4) permit manipulation (synthesis and analysis) of the speech sounds, and (5) help the subject apply this knowledge for rapid and precise speech decoding. The therapy methods were based, in part, on those suggested by DiCarlo (1957) and Winitz (1971).

General Considerations

In order to encode a clear, robust phonemic message, slow, clear speech was used by the clinicians. Phonemic stimulation was carried out in quiet therapy rooms or in audiometric test chambers, whenever possible. For patient 2 (Carol), the signal was improved by saying the sounds directly into the auxiliary microphone held in front of the clinician's mouth. Visual cues were given only when required (e.g., for instructions). Variation in the presentation of individual sounds was minimized. All sounds were given in the stressed, neutral (not coarticulated) positions.

Repetition is an important feature of this therapy. Unlike cognitive therapy that deals with ideas (in which a single presentation may be sufficient), reteaching the brain what these many phonemes sound like is a very different matter. This is a difficult task for the patient because it requires careful analysis and memory for these brief, complex sounds. Perceptions must be narrowed to a finer and finer degree as new sounds are added in competition. Unlike a normal listener who has a clear perception of sounds, the person who was formerly deaf has only a vague and obsolete concept that is not easily improved, except with repetition and structured listening.

The positioning of graphic materials was frequently changed to maintain alertness and avoid confusions. For the same reason, the same combination of sounds was not given repeatedly at one time. Therapy always progressed from easier to harder tasks; we preferred going too slowly rather than moving ahead too quickly.

Initially, phonemic therapy was provided at least two times a week because perception of some sounds was so weak that the new images were not maintained long. Sessions were generally one hour in length. Longer sessions were not profitable because the therapy was quite fatiguing for the patients. Eight steps used in the therapy are described next. Repetition and review of these steps was essential at succeeding sessions and during the same session.

Introduction of Phonemes

Phonemes were taught, one at a time, using a four-stage approach, as follows:

1. Without revealing the phoneme, a sound was repeated three or four times, using an irregular cadence (e.g., /b..b...b/).
2. The sound was identified for the subject when it was said a few more times with the clinician's lips visable.
3. The patient was then told, "The sound is /b/ as in *book, boy, baby,* and *tub.*" Quite often, the patient was surprised at which sound it turned out to be.
4. The final step in introducing phonemes was to associate the sound with a letter printed on a small card—in this case, the letter *B*. Each time the sound was said, the patient was to point to the card (always correctly because, at this point, there was only one card to choose from).

Discrimination

The discrimination phase was used to help the subject differentiate two to perhaps six sounds, with enough repetition to assist the person's memory. We started with only one sound—for example, the /b/ sound with the *B* card in front of the patient. After a few repetitions, a second (previously introduced) sound was presented (e.g., /s/). With two cards showing, the sounds were presented (e.g., /b...s..s....b/), with the patient pointing to the appropriate card. After a few more presentations, the position of the cards was varied in some way. Then another sound that had been introduced previously was added (e.g., /b....r...s..r/).

Easy distinctions were used at first. Unfortunately, the confusions of normal hearers or hearing-impaired listeners are not necessarily the same as the ones we found in patients with CIs. For example, n/v, t/tʃ and o/l confusions were common (although o/l is also seen in CAP decoding cases).

Focusing of Attenuation

During the discrimination phase, patients often had difficulty distinguishing between two or more sounds. One subject stated emphatically that there is no difference between the /s/ and /ʃ/ sounds. One can bring out the differences by stimulating with one sound several times (irregular cadence) and then presenting the other sound (e.g., /s...s...s..s.... s.s..ʃ/). This generally made the differences more salient, but the subjects were unable to maintain the distinction with a single series. Additional repetitions of the series, with review at subsequent visits, proved helpful.

Short-Term Memory

It is surprising how short memory is for some newly acquired sounds. In a minute or two, these patients may forget the sensation that constitutes a sound. Exercises were useful for improving retention. The patient was encouraged to keep the sound clearly in mind. Several cards were shown from which one sound was spoken. The patient was not to respond immediately to the sound, but rather to wait for a signal from the clinician before responding. Once that task was mastered, the cards remained covered until a response was requested. Longer and longer delays were used and eventually the cards were omitted.

Interference Memory

It was noted that the introduction of a second sound often obliterated memory for the first. Thus, after short-term memory was strengthened, we sought to improve interference memory. From a group of perhaps six cards, two of them were sounded (separated by a pause). The patient was asked to point to both cards or, later, to say the sounds. In time, the cards were concealed until the response was requested. When the patient became proficient with the previous steps, the person was asked to say the two sounds without benefit of cards.

The interference memory task was expanded to introduce phonemic synthesis. For example, a column of four consonant cards was arranged next to a column of four vowel cards. Sounds such as /s . . . o/ or /b . . . i/ were given. When the patient repeated the two sounds correctly, he or she was asked, "Can you put the sounds together to form a word?" If not, instruction was given on how to combine the sounds and the same combinations were tried again. Instead of interfering with one another, the sounds could now cling to one another and actually simplify the task of remembering them.

Phonemic Synthesis (PS)

Phonemic synthesis (PS) is the process of combining a sound with the next one(s) until all the sounds can be formed into a word (or nonsense word). Phonemes were given at a rate of one-per-second *or slower.* Three columns of sound cards (consonants, vowels, and consonants) were set before the person as an aid. Two or three sounds were said (e.g., going from the left column to the right, /s . . . o . . . p/ = soap) and the patient was to provide the word. As in other tasks, we eventually worked toward open-set performance.

Although PS is often the starting point for auditory training with those who have a CAPD, it took perhaps 10 visits before our prelingually deafened patients were able to carry out this task, and then only with the aid of cards (which are not needed for people with CAP problems). PS is extremely important. Often, the patients made important observations about words or sounds during this task, as it relates component sounds to words.

Phonemic Analysis

Phonemic analysis is the opposite of PS, and more difficult. The patient is given a word and must divide it into its component sounds. At first, we employed words that had been used in PS activities. This was the first task in the therapy program in which the patient had to decode words rather than sounds.

Other Speech Tasks

We believe, given improved phonemic skills, most patients will be able to incorporate this understanding for decoding speech. However, to ensure optimal benefit, some work was geared to bridging the gap. One method used lists of names that the patient encountered. These lists included names of family, friends, and colleagues. After obtaining baseline with 36 names, we began working on subsets of 12, one at a time. The ones that received the most attention improved the greatest. The names that created the most confusions were treated either as discrimination tasks or were targeted for focused attention practice (described earlier), using cards with the names on them (instead of the individual phonemes).

In time, predictable sentences were given using these names (e.g., "Is Ben your uncle in Los Angeles?" "Is Elizabeth your childhood friend from second grade?"). Reading how-to-do-it books on topics known to the patient was found to be an easy way to introduce paragraphs and related sentences.

THERAPEUTIC RESULTS

Jack, who had performed quite well on the pretests, quickly demonstrated improvement on the PRT retests. Within three weeks, he was using the telephone in situations in which he previously was unable to do. Carol had performed close to chance initially, with only a few sounds inconsistently correct on PRT and no words correct on WRS. However, Carol gradually improved over time and has continued to do so during the year of therapy. After one month of therapy, Carol was using the telephone.

It should be noted that there was some variability in test performance. This was due to fatigue and other unknown or unavoidable factors, including equipment problems and the need for remapping. Score
differences due to testers was rare and, when noted, accounted for no
more than a few percentage points.

Jack's PRT scores are shown in Figure 13.3. It can be seen that he
began at about the 40 percent point, which is most impressive for a prelingually deaf person. His scores improved until he reached 100 percent
(11 months later) and then leveled off to about the 85 percent range
(although the most recent tests were administered during a period when
he had little or no therapy). His WRSs for words and sounds are shown
in Figure 13.4. Although little work was directed toward words or sentences, Jack was able to apply his improved decoding skills to these
longer units of speech. He scored 100 percent on the CID Every Day Sentences (auditory only).

**Figure 13.3   Phoneme Recognition Test Scores (in percent correct)
for Subject 1 (Jack), from January 1995 to August 1996**

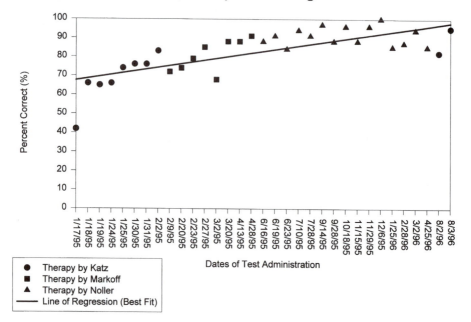

**Figure 13.4   Word Recognition Scores (in percent correct) *(A)* for
Words and *(B)* Component Sounds of These Words for Subject 1 (Jack)**

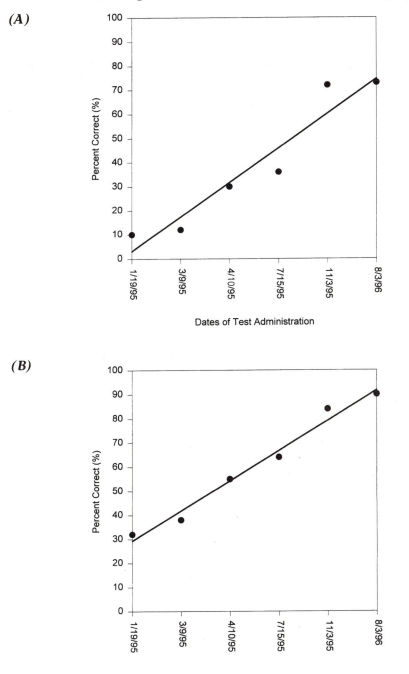

(A)

Percent Correct (%)

Dates of Test Administration

(B)

Percent Correct (%)

Dates of Test Administration

Carol's PRT scores are shown in Figure 13.5. Her first score shown was 20 percent correct; however, this was not a pretherapy baseline. Her two previous scores were much poorer, but are not shown because they were recorded tests. Despite variations, Carol has continued to improve gradually over time, despite her very limited performance initially. After 20 visits, she reached the level at which Jack was performing initially. She is now scoring at about the 70 percent level, although most of these tests were given following a four-month hiatus from therapy. Figure 13.6 shows Carol's WRSs for words and sounds and Figure 13.7 depicts her CID Every Day Sentence scores. It should be noted that we had no baseline for her sentence abilities, as she was first given this test after more than six months of therapy.

Figure 13.5   Phoneme Recognition Test Scores, (in percent correct) for Subject 2 (Carol), from September 1995 to August 1996

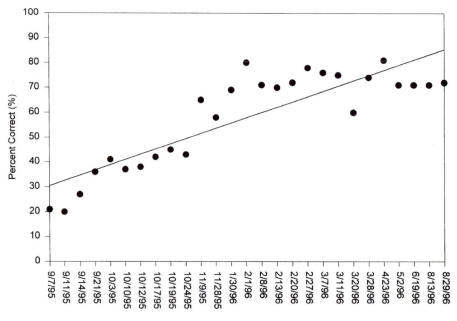

Dates of Test Administration

Figure 13.6   Word Recognition Scores (in percent correct) (A) for Words and (B) Component Sounds of These Words for Subject 2 (Carol)

(A)

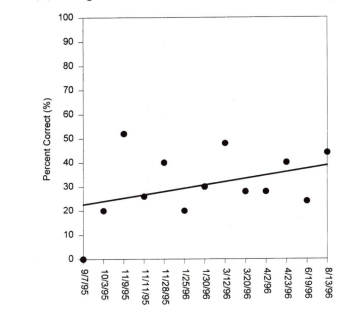

Dates of Test Administration

(B)

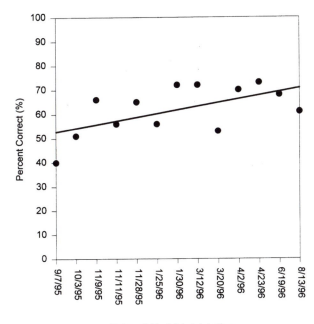

Dates of Test Administration

FIGURE 13.7 CID Everyday Sentences (in percent of words correct) for Subject 2 (Carol). There was no baseline information for this procedure, as the first test was given six months after therapy had begun.

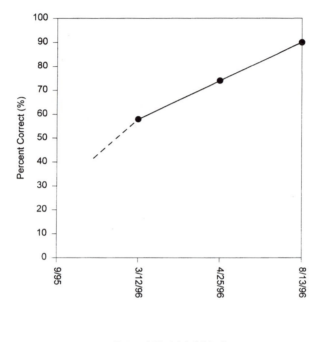

Dates of Test Administration

DISCUSSION

Our experience with CAP therapy for patients with CIs has been highly positive and more successful than anticipated. Both of these individuals with prelingual deafness made considerable gains in their test scores and in their everyday performance. When sounds were used in therapy, the individuals tended to improve on them, and when sounds were not worked on, performance on the sounds tended to remain unchanged. However, later on in therapy, as they improved further, even some of the nontreated sounds began to improve as well.

For Carol, after three months we had worked on nearly half of the consonant sounds and took this opportunity to compare performance before and after therapy for the "treated" and "nontreated" sounds. On the nine sounds that were worked on in therapy, she improved by 34 percent, but on the non-treated sounds, she improved by only 5 percent.

We can also look at the quality of errors, which improved from gross errors to refined ones. Table 13.1 shows the responses that Carol made when given the PRT the first 10 times (a total of 20 presentation for each phoneme in different scramblings). Initially, there were confusions between consonant and vowel sounds. For example, when the /h/ was given, she once called it an /ɛ/ and once /ak/. These were among the 13 sounds, or sound combinations, that she confused with the /h/. For the 20 trials, she failed to get it correct even once. After seven months of therapy, her last 10 PRTs showed 70 percent accuracy for /h/, and the errors that she did make were quite reasonable. They were /k, f, p/.

Both Jack and Carol have indicated that when they are not in therapy for a period of months, they feel their skills decreasing somewhat. This reduction in their mental image of sounds has not caused a major change in their PRT to date, especially after a few therapy sessions. In general, our experience suggests that intensive therapy initially is important to develop a good basis for phonemic decoding. Two sessions a week for one hour each is recommended. After six months or so, as skills

TABLE 13.1 Phoneme Recognition Test Responses for Subject 2 (Carol): First 10 Times Tested vs. 7 Months Later

Sound Presented	Response Errors	Percent Correct
Initial Responses on PRT (First 10 Times Tested)		
b	i, d, I, g, p, k	20
s	ks, e, n, sk, o en, ʃ,tʃ	30
h	f, ks, k, I, b, ak θ, t, p, g, ʌ, ɛ, ʃ	0
d	I, f, i, p, t, k, g b, ɛ	0
z	l, au, æ,ʃ, u, a, h, e, s	0
Final Responses on PRT (10 Times Tested After 7 Months of Therapy)		
b	(no errors)	100
s	ʃ, f, h	75
h	k, f, p	70
d	g	65
z	s, v	70

become stronger, less concentrated therapy is sufficient to maintain the benefits and to correct the misconceptions that occur. During the early stages, sporadic therapy does not appear to be very effective.

We are in the early stages of our work on CAP therapy for patients with CIs. Thus far, we have had limited opportunities to work with children and postlingually deafened adults. We are also interested in the long-term benefits of therapy for Jack and Carol, and to see what effects, if any, the therapy has on speech production.

REFERENCES

DiCarlo, L. M. (1957). Personal communication.

Katz, J. (1983). Phonemic synthesis. In E. Lasky, & J. Katz, (Eds.), *Central auditory processing disorders: Problems of speech, language and learning* (pp. 269–296). Baltimore: University Park Press.

Katz, J. (1992). Classification of auditory processing disorders. In J. Katz, N. Stecker, & D. Henderson (Eds.), *Central auditory processing: A transdisciplinary view* (pp. 81–92). St. Louis: Mosby-Yearbook.

Katz, J., & Burge, C. (1971). Auditory perception training for children with learning disabilities. *Menorah Medical J., 2,* 18–29.

Katz, J., & Medol, E. (1972). The use of phonemic synthesis in speech therapy. *Menorah Medical J., 3,* 10–13.

Katz, J., & Smith, P. S. (1991). A ten minute look at the CNS through the ears: Using the SSW test. In R. Zappula et al. (Eds.), Windows on the brain: Neuropsychologies technical frontiers. *Ann NY Acad Sci, 620,* 233–251.

Lasky, E. Z., & Katz, J. (1983). *Central auditory processing disorders: Problems of speech, language and learning* (p. 5). Baltimore: University Park Press.

NIH Consensus Statement. (1995). Cochlear implants in adults and children. *National Institutes of Health, 13*(2), 1–30.

Osberger, M. J. (1990). Audiological rehabilitation with cochlear implants and tactile aids. *Asha, 32,* 38–43.

Parkin, J. L., & Dankowski, M. K. (1986). Speech performance by patients with multichannel cochlear implants. *Otolaryngology, Head, and Neck Surgery, 95,* 205–209.

Winitz, H. (1971). Personal communication.

ACKNOWLEDGMENTS

I would like to express my appreciation to Jack King, Carol Marie Kraus, Katie Noller, Lori Markoff, Patti Trautwein, and Amy Nostrant.

AUTHOR INDEX

SUBJECT INDEX

Phoneme Recognition Test (PRT), 221,
 225–226, 228–229, 231
Phonemic analysis, 225
Phonemic Synthesis (PS) Test, 3, 5, 6, 7,
 8, 17, 109, 156, 161, 162
Phonemic synthesis therapy, 17, 18,
 224–225, 152
Phonemic therapy procedures,
 222–225
 discrimination, 223
 focusing attention, 223
 general considerations, 222
 interference memory, 224
 introduction of phonemes, 223
 other speech tasks, 225
 phonemic analysis, 225
 phonemic synthesis, 224
 short-term memory, 224
Phonemic training, 218–219, 222–232
Plasticity, 18, 19, 152
 compensatory, 19
 developmental, 19
 learning-related, 19
 neural, 152
Pragmatics, 80
Preferential seating, 77, 123, 126
Prelingually deaf, 218–220
Progressive Matrices Test, 157–159,
 161–163
PSI sentences, 96

Reading comprehension, 50
Receptive language skills, 5, 6, 8
Reciprocal teaching, 56
Rehearsal, 70, 82–83, 124, 144
Remediation techniques, 91
Repetition, 222
Reverberation, 89, 90

Reversals, 8
RNA, 23

Schema, 70
Self-advocacy, 57–58, 112–113,
 208–209
Self-control, 55, 57
Self-esteem, 56
Self-regulation, 52
Signal-to-noise (S/N) ratio, 90, 91, 92,
 100, 109
Sound field FM systems, 91, 93, 94, 106
Sound localization, 24
Speech-in-noise, desensitization, 152
Speech-in-noise test, 3, 5, 6, 7, 8, 153,
 156, 161, 162
Speech-language evaluation, 4, 5
Speech sound discrimination, 18
SPIN sentences, 96
Staggered Spondaic Word (SSW) Test,
 3, 5, 6, 7, 8, 92, 93, 153, 156,
 158, 160–162, 167
Synthetic approach to auditory
 training (*see* Auditory training)

Temporal processing, 91
Time-altered speech test, 153
Time-expanded speech, 18
Tolerance-fading memory (TFM), 5, 9,
 10, 11, 118, 217, 123

WIPI words, 96
Word-finding difficulty, 5, 119
Word-finding test, 4
Word recognition, 18, 216–218
 open set, 216–218
Word recognition/discrimination test,
 221, 225–227